# 100 Questions & Answers About Congestive Heart Failure

Campion Quinn, MD, MHA
Internist and Medical Consultant
Rockville Centre, NY

**JONES AND BARTLETT PUBLISHERS**
*Sudbury, Massachusetts*
BOSTO͏ LONDON SINGAPORE

D1427062

*World Headquarters*
Jones and Bartlett
Publishers
40 Tall Pine Drive
Sudbury, MA 01776
info@jbpub.com
www.jbpub.com

Jones and Bartlett
Publishers Canada
2406 Nikanna Road
Mississauga, ON L5C
2W6
CANADA

Jones and Bartlett
Publishers International
Barb House, Barb Mews
London W6 7PA
UK

Jones and Bartlett's books and products are available through most bookstores and online booksellers. To contact Jones and Bartlett Publishers directly, call 800-832-0034, fax 978-443-8000, or visit our website www.jbpub.com.

Substantial discounts on bulk quantities of Jones and Bartlett's publications are available to corporations, professional associations, and other qualified organizations. For details and specific discount information, contact the special sales department at Jones and Bartlett via the above contact information or send an email to specialsales@jbpub.com.

Copyright © 2006 by Jones and Bartlett Publishers, Inc.

All rights reserved. No part of the material protected by this copyright notice may be reproduced or utilized in any form, electronic or mechanical, including photocopying, recording, or by any information storage and retrieval system, without written permission from the copyright owner.

**Library of Congress Cataloging-in-Publication Data**
Quinn, Campion E.
  100 questions and answers about congestive heart failure / Campion E. Quinn.
    p. cm.
Includes index.
  ISBN 0-7637-3897-2
1. Congestive heart failure. 2. Congestive heart failure—Miscellanea. I. Title: One hundred questions and answers about congestive heart failure. II. Title.
  RC685.C53Q85 2005
  616.1'29—dc22

                                                                2005021186
                                                                6048

**Production Credits**

Executive Publisher: Christopher Davis
Associate Editor: Kathy Richardson
Production Editor: Karen Ferreira
Associate Marketing Manager: Laura Kavigian
Cover Design: Philip Regan

Manufacturing Buyer: Therese Connell
Composition: Modern Graphics
Printing and Binding: Malloy Lithographing
Cover Printer: Malloy Lithographing

The authors, editor, and publisher have made every effort to provide accurate information. However, they are not responsible for errors, omissions, or for any outcomes related to the use of the contents of this book and take no responsibility for the use of the products described. Treatments and side effects described in this book may not be applicable to all patients; likewise, some patients may require a dose or experience a side effect that is not described herein. The reader should confer with his or her own physician regarding specific treatments and side effects. Drugs and medical devices are discussed that may have limited availability controlled by the Food and Drug Administration (FDA) for use only in a research study or clinical trial. The drug information presented has been derived from reference sources, recently published data, and pharmaceutical research data. Research, clinical practice, and government regulations often change the accepted standard in this field. When consideration is being given to use of any drug in the clinical setting, the health care provider or reader is responsible for determining FDA status of the drug, reading the package insert, reviewing prescribing information for the most up-to-date recommendations on dose, precautions, and contraindications, and determining the appropriate usage for the product. This is especially important in the case of drugs that are new or seldom used.

Printed in the United States of America

09 08 07 06 05   10 9 8 7 6 5 4 3 2 1

*For My Mother,*
*Maureen Quinn,*
*who continues to raise her 13 children,*
*no matter how old we get.*

| ROCHDALE LIBRARIES | |
| --- | --- |
| 616·129 Q41 | |
| 1200943 | |
| Bertrams | 22.06.06 |
| | £12.99 |
| | |

Congestive heart failure (CHF) is a common disease and it is becoming more common by the day. Current medical technology prevents many more cardiac deaths than before. However, this boon comes at a cost. The cost is more patients surviving with CHF. CHF is a serious illness that can leave its victims fatigued, short of breath, and unable to work. Although there is no cure for CHF, there are effective treatments.

Medical studies have shown that CHF patients who are well informed about their disease and who understand their treatment regimen fair better than those who do not. These well-informed patients adhere more closely to their treatment regimens, have fewer visits to the hospital, and have better outcomes than the patients who are not well informed.

Although physicians know how to diagnose and treat CHF patients, the patient is often unprepared to assume a role in his or her own care because of a lack of medical information. Traditionally, providing medical information was the role of the primary care physician who had the medical training, the available time, and a well-developed relationship with the patient. Unfortunately, this is often not the case today.

Today, there are more tests, more treatments, and more choices than ever before—yet there is less time to explain them and frankly, many physicians lack the communication skills necessary to explain the vast amount of information about CHF and its treatment in a way that is accessible to their patients. To compound this problem, physicians have less time to spend with each patient. Still, more patient education is needed.

This book is a good start at filling that need. Information and advice are offered on many of the most important topics in CHF, including the questions, fears, and frustrations that patients commonly bring to their doctor. While avoiding oversimplification, clear and medically accurate explanations are offered. Complex clinical topics are explained using everyday language. Important medical terms are fully defined. The glossary of medical terms is an excellent tool for looking up unfamiliar terms and the appendix provides many resources for information and support of the CHF patient.

For a CHF patient and their loved ones, dealing with a diagnosis of CHF can be frightening and getting accurate information can be daunting. There are new tests, new medicines, and many important choices to be made. The right information can ease anxiety and make choices simpler. This well-organized and easy-to-read book will answer many of your questions, decrease your anxiety, and help you to stay healthy.

**Ali R. Homayuni, MD, FACC, FSCAI, FACP**
Clinical Associate Professor of Medicine and Cardiology
State University of New York,
Downstate Medical College, Brooklyn, New York
Associate Director of Interventional Cardiology
The Staten Island University Hospital
Staten Island, New York

I wrote this book for the patient with congestive heart disease and their family. It is my hope that this book will provide useful information about congestive heart disease and that it will help the patient to live a healthier and more comfortable life.

Although this book can be read from cover to cover, it was designed as a reference text, so that a patient or caregiver can review particular questions and answers that are immediately important.

This book is not comprehensive in its scope and only deals with the most frequently asked questions, in order to explore them in as much detail as possible.

# PART ONE

# The Basics

What is congestive heart failure (CHF)?

Is CHF serious?

Is there a cure for heart failure?

*More . . .*

# 1. What is congestive heart failure?

The term **congestive heart failure (CHF)** is used interchangeably with the term **heart failure**; they both indicate the same condition. Heart failure is a condition that results from the inability of the heart to pump blood effectively to the rest of the body or the heart requires a higher filling pressure in order to pump effectively. Put simply, heart failure means that your heart can't pump enough blood to keep all your body's tissues and organs working properly.

It is important to note that the definition of congestive heart failure does not identify any particular problem with the heart or blood vessels. That is because heart failure itself is not a disease, but develops as a result of other conditions that damage the heart. Common conditions that can damage the heart include:

- Long-term, untreated high blood pressure
- **Coronary artery disease**
- **Heart attack**
- Diseases of heart muscle itself (**cardiomyopathy**)
- Viral infections of the heart muscle (**myocarditis**)
- Toxins that affect the heart muscle (such as some chemotherapy agents)
- Diseases of the **heart valves (endocarditis)**

Sometimes CHF develops quickly, over days to weeks, but most often congestive heart failure develops slowly, as the heart gradually weakens and has more difficulty keeping up with its workload.

Heart failure may range in severity from a moderate decrease in function without any symptoms to significant damage that leaves a person seriously weakened and very symptomatic. Although heart failure is a seri-

## Sidebar definitions

**Congestive heart failure (CHF)**

A common form of heart failure that causes swelling and fluid retention in the legs and ankles and congestion in the lungs.

**Heart failure**

An illness in which the heart doesn't pump blood through the body as it should. Heart failure has no cure, but it can be treated with medications, diet, and other lifestyle changes.

**Coronary artery disease**

A condition in which the arteries that supply blood to the heart muscle become blocked. Less oxygen-rich blood can flow to the heart, making it weak. Severe cases can result in heart attack.

**Heart attack**

Sudden death of a section of the heart muscle caused by a decrease in blood supply to that area.

ous condition, much can be done to manage its effects and its impact on a patient's life.

Heart failure is a term that is frequently misused, especially when given as a cause of death. Heart failure is not synonymous with "cessation of heartbeat"; rather it implies an inability of the heart to keep up with the demands of the body.

Victoria's comment:

*I've been a CHF patient for more than 8 years. The doctor said I had high blood pressure and coronary artery disease for many years that led up to the development of CHF.*

## 2. Is CHF common?

According to the American Heart Association, nearly 5 million people experience heart failure and about 550,000 new cases are diagnosed each year in the United States. Heart failure becomes more prevalent with age. The condition affects 1 percent of people aged 50 years and older and about 5 percent of those aged 75 years and older. In fact, heart failure is the commonest reason for admission to a hospital for people 65 and over.

African-Americans experience heart failure twice as often as Caucasians and are 1.5 times more likely to die of CHF than whites are. Nevertheless, African-American patients appear to have similar or lower in-hospital mortality rates than white patients.

Between the ages of 40 to 75, men experience heart failure more than women. However, after the age of 75, women catch up and the difference between the sexes disappears.

**Cardiomyopathy**
A disease of the heart muscle, it has many causes.

**Myocarditis**
An inflammation of the heart muscle. Myocarditis is an uncommon disorder caused by viral infections such as coxsackie virus, adenovirus, and echovirus. It may also occur during or after various viral, bacterial, or parasitic infections.

**Heart valves**
Structures in the heart that open and close with each heartbeat. The heart has four valves that work together to control the flow of blood through the heart and body.

**Endocarditis**
An infection, commonly bacterial, that occurs on the inner lining of the heart and heart valves.

*CHF is among the most serious diseases in the United States today.*

Health experts at the National Institutes of Health (NIH) expect these numbers to grow even more for two main reasons. The first is that cardiac patients are now able to survive and live longer with their disease because of more effective treatments. This increases their chances of developing CHF. The second reason is that the elderly population continues to grow as a percentage of the overall population, making it likely that the number of people with heart failure will increase as well.

## 3. Is CHF serious?

Yes, CHF is among the most serious diseases in the United States today. The fatigue and shortness of breath associated with CHF can be very debilitating, leaving some patients unable to perform even their activities of daily living such as cooking, cleaning, and grooming themselves. This level of disability severely affects their quality of life.

CHF affects nearly 5 million Americans, with more than 550,000 new cases diagnosed each year. Significantly, the number of patients with CHF is growing. In the past 5 years, the Medicare program has reported a 5 percent annual increase in the number of patients with this diagnosis. With 80 percent of hospitalizations occurring in individuals older than 65 years and 50 percent in patients older than 75 years, CHF is the most frequently reported diagnosis in Medicare patients.

There are two prominent reasons for the increased incidence of CHF: the aging population and modern medical care. More effective medical treatments for heart attacks have decreased the mortality rates. The survivors of these heart attacks comprise a rapidly growing group of younger patients with CHF. The aging of the population creates a greater number of people who have risk factors for CHF, such as chronic high blood pressure, diabetes, and coronary artery disease.

CHF is an important cause of sickness and results in frequent doctor and hospital visits. These visits consume an enormous amount of health care resources. CHF is the most common indication for admission to the hospital among older persons. Patients, insurers, and health care agencies spent an estimated $20 billion in 2003 for the care of CHF patients. This includes costs related to hospital care, office visits, home care, long-term care, and medications. CHF is the single most costly health care problem in the United States and the second leading reason for hospitalization in patients over 65 years of age. CHF costs exceed those for treating **myocardial infarctions (MIs)** and cancers combined.

**Myocardial infarction (MI)**
Another term for heart attack.

CHF can result in death. It accounts for more than a quarter of a million deaths in this country and is the most common cause of death in people over 65.

Although heart failure produces extremely high mortality rates, specific treatments, particularly **beta blockers** and devices that stabilize heart rhythms, are now dramatically improving survival rates in patients with severe heart failure.

**Beta blockers**
Medications that keep the heart rate from increasing in response to stress. Beta blockers are used in the treatment of high blood pressure (hypertension). Some beta blockers are also used to relieve angina (chest pain) and in heart attack patients to help prevent additional heart attacks. Beta blockers are also used to correct irregular heartbeats.

Victoria's comment:

*When I was first diagnosed with CHF, I was admitted to the hospital four times in the same year with shortness of breath and leg swelling. It seemed I was always short of breath and couldn't go outside at all without spending the next day in bed. I eventually got on the right medications and really started to watch my salt intake. Now I haven't been admitted to the hospital in more than 3 years.*

# 4. Are all CHF patients the same?

No, not all CHF patients are the same. Some are sicker and require more treatment than others. When treating patients, physicians need to be able to identify how severe a patient's CHF is. For this reason, many CHF classification systems were developed. These classifications help physicians determine what a patient's treatment plan should be. The most widely used classification system for CHF is the **New York Heart Association (NYHA) classification** system. According to this system, a patient's heart failure is rated on a scale of I to IV with "Class I" patients having the mildest symptoms and "Class IV" patients having the worst. (See table.)

Only about 5 percent of patients have extremely severe Class IV heart failure. However, as an overall statistic,

**New York Heart Association (NYHA) classification**

A classification scheme in which a patient's CHF symptoms are divided into four levels of severity.

**Palpitations**

Rapid or irregular heartbeats.

**Table 1    The NYHA Classification System for Heart Failure**

| The NYHA Classification of Heart Failure | |
|---|---|
| **Class I** | The patient has no limitation of physical activity. He or she experiences no shortness of breath, fatigue, or heart **palpitations** with ordinary physical activity |
| **Class II** | The patient has slight limitation of physical activity. He or she has shortness of breath, fatigue, or heart palpitations with ordinary physical activity, but is comfortable at rest. |
| **Class III** | The patient experiences marked limitation of activity. Shortness of breath, fatigue, or heart palpitations with *less than* ordinary physical activity, but the patient is comfortable at rest. |
| **Class IV** | The patient suffers from severe to complete limitation of activity. Shortness of breath, fatigue, or heart palpitations with *any* physical exertion and symptoms appear even at rest. |

only 30 to 50 percent of these patients are alive 5 years after the diagnosis is made.

The NYHA classification system is very useful for doctors and nurses who treat patients with heart failure. It helps patients and doctors tell if heart failure is improving, staying the same, or getting worse. It is also used in research studies to help tell if treatments are successful. The NYHA classification system is used worldwide.

It must be emphasized that these classification methods aren't perfect as predictors of how CHF will progress or how a patient will respond to medications. The biggest problem is that a patient's symptoms may not always relate to the actual severity of his or her condition. In fact, one study found that half of heart failure patients who complained of breathlessness after exercise had only mild heart abnormalities. Another confounding factor is that some patients do not report fatigue or shortness of breath after physical activity and yet they may have severe heart damage. Experts suggest that physicians be sure to consider other factors that may indicate a poorer outlook and require aggressive treatments.

## 5. Is CHF different for different ethnic groups?

Yes, different ethnic groups appear to have different incidences of CHF. Further, different ethnic groups appear to use medical services at different rates.

For example, studies indicate that African-Americans suffer a disproportionate incidence of cardiovascular disease. With respect to heart failure, they are affected

*Different ethnic groups appear to have different incidences of CHF.*

The Basics

at a rate almost twice the rate of the corresponding white population and are more likely to die from it at a younger age. This dramatic ethnic difference in health outcomes has been attributed to a variety of factors, including access to medical care, management of heart failure, and socioeconomic factors. Recent analyses of heart failure clinical trials, however, show that the mortality rate and the hospitalization rate for African-Americans is significantly higher than that of non-African-Americans, even after adjustment for such factors. In fact, black heart-failure patients also have different morbidity and mortality than do whites, dying at a rate 40–50 percent faster than the corresponding white population.

**Angiotensin**

Any of several vaso-constrictor sub-stances that cause narrowing of blood vessels.

There are clinical data that suggest that hypertension in African-Americans is less well controlled with **angiotensin**-converting-enzyme (ACE) inhibitor therapy. Thus, different medication regimens may be necessary to control this disease in African-Americans. (See the medication BiDil in question number 47.)

When compared to other ethnic groups, African-Americans had the highest rate of CHF hospitalization. Age-adjusted hospitalization rates were comparable among whites, Latinos, and Asian women and all were lower than those for African-Americans. Overall, Asian men had the lowest rates. On adjusted analyses, African-Americans were more likely than whites and Asians to be rehospitalized.

Based on data from the U.S. Census Bureau and the Centers for Disease Control and Prevention, scientists estimate that 750,000 African-Americans have been diagnosed with heart failure. They expect this number to grow to approximately 900,000 persons by 2010.

## 6. How quickly does heart failure develop?

Heart failure is usually a chronic disease. That means it's a long-term condition that tends to become worse gradually. By the time someone is diagnosed, chances are that the heart has been losing pumping capacity little by little for quite a while. At first the heart tries to make up for this by:

- Enlarging. When the heart chamber enlarges, it stretches more and can contract more strongly, so it pumps more blood.
- Developing more muscle mass. The increase in muscle mass occurs because the contracting cells of the heart get bigger. This allows the heart to pump more forcefully, at least initially.
- Pumping faster. This helps to increase the heart's output.

The body also tries to compensate in other ways. The blood vessels narrow to keep blood pressure up, trying to make up for the heart's loss of power. The body diverts blood away from less important tissues and organs to maintain flow to the most vital organs, the heart and brain. These temporary measures mask the problem of heart failure, but they don't solve it. This helps explain why some people may not become aware of their condition until years after their heart begins its decline. (It's also a good reason to have regular checkups with your doctor.) Eventually the heart and body just can't keep up and the person experiences the

The Basics

*Because heart
failure is not a
disease, it
can't really be
"cured."*

fatigue, breathing problems, or other symptoms that usually prompt a trip to the doctor.

Victoria's comment:

*My cardiologist told me years before I was first diagnosed that I would develop heart failure if I didn't control my weight and blood pressure. I had high blood pressure for 22 years before I first noticed that I was getting short of breath.*

## 7. Is there a cure for heart failure?

The short answer is no. Congestive heart failure is a condition that is a collection of signs and symptoms. Because heart failure is not a disease, it can't really be "cured," although this doesn't mean that CHF can't be successfully treated. In some cases, heart failure can even be completely reversed, although this is less common. Treatment of underlying causative factors such as low thyroid hormone or blocked coronary arteries and reducing risk factors such as high blood pressure, smoking, and alcohol intake can make a big difference in treating or reversing the symptoms of congestive heart failure.

### The Heart and How It Works

Before further discussing congestive heart failure, it is important to briefly review the basic make-up of the heart and how it works to circulate your blood.

The heart is a muscular organ in the middle of your chest. It is approximately the size of your clenched fist and it is the "pump" that circulates all the blood in your body. The contractions of this muscular pump are the heartbeats you can feel and that your doctor listens to with a stethoscope.

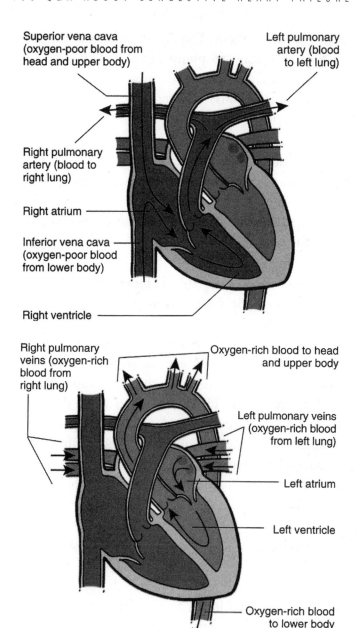

Superior vena cava
(oxygen-poor blood from
head and upper body)

Left pulmonary
artery (blood
to left lung)

Right pulmonary
artery (blood to
right lung)

Right atrium

Inferior vena cava
(oxygen-poor blood
from lower body)

Right ventricle

Right pulmonary
veins (oxygen-rich
blood from
right lung)

Oxygen-rich blood to head
and upper body

Left pulmonary veins
(oxygen-rich blood
from left lung)

Left atrium

Left ventricle

Oxygen-rich blood
to lower body

**Figure 1   Heart anatomy.**

The heart is divided into four chambers. There are two atria and two ventricles. The atria, which are located at the top of the heart, are smaller and have thinner walls. The atria are connected to the

**Atria**

The upper two chambers of the heart.

*The Basics*

*13*

*The heart is divided into four chambers.*

ventricles below them. The atrium and ventricle work together as a team to pump blood out of the heart. Although they are connected to each other, each one of the two sets of atria and ventricles pumps blood to a different place.

The right atrium and ventricle take blood from the largest vein in the body (the vena cava) and pump it into the lungs for oxygenation. The left atrium and ventricle take blood coming from the lungs and pump it into the rest of the body.

When your blood circulates, it moves blood from the veins in your body toward your heart. This blood in your veins is low in oxygen and high in carbon dioxide. The blood enters the right upper chamber of your heart, the right **atrium**. When the atrium contracts, the blood is moved into the larger chamber below it called the right **ventricle**. Here, the blood from the veins, which is filled with carbon dioxide, is propelled into the lungs. The lungs are able to get rid of the carbon dioxide and put oxygen into the blood. This oxygenated blood circulates out of the lungs and into the left side of the heart.

The blood from the lungs enters the left atrium and when this chamber contracts, it pushes the blood into the largest chamber of the heart, the left ventricle. The left ventricle's job is to push the blood into the **aorta**, the largest artery in the body. Because this chamber supplies most of the heart's pumping power, it's larger and has more muscle mass than the other chambers. From the aorta, the blood circulates to all the organs of the body, bringing oxygen and carrying away carbon dioxide.

**Atrium**

An upper chamber of the heart, called atria in the plural.

**Ventricle**

One of the two larger chambers of the heart. The ventricles sit below the atria in the heart.

**Aorta**

The largest artery in the body. It leads from the top of the heart and travels down the chest into the abdomen with branches to arms, legs, and all major organs.

## 8. What causes heart failure?

All of the risk factors for heart disease also increase the risk for heart failure. Heart failure results from other diseases and conditions that damage the heart. If untreated, any one of these conditions can damage the heart and lead to heart failure. Patients who have more than one condition face an even greater risk of developing failure.

These conditions include:

**High blood pressure (hypertension)** In high blood pressure, the pressure and resistance in the body's arteries is increased. As a result, the heart must work harder to pump blood against this elevated pressure and into the arteries. This increased workload can, over time, lead to an enlarged and poorly functioning heart.

**Diabetes** In some cases, diabetes seems to cause damage to the heart muscle, increasing the likelihood that heart failure will develop. In addition, patients with diabetes have other risk factors for coronary heart disease and therefore may be at an increased risk for developing heart failure. (See below.)

**Coronary heart disease** When the arteries to the heart muscle (coronary arteries) become narrowed due to cholesterol deposits, the blood flow to the heart is decreased. When the heart muscle doesn't get enough blood and oxygen (especially during exercise, when the body needs more blood supply and oxygen), the heart does not pump as well. This can result in fatigue and shortness of breath. If enough of the coronary arteries are affected, the heart muscles will not have enough blood supply to pump adequately, and the heart will go into failure.

*The Basics*

If the decrease in blood supply to the heart muscle is critical, it can result in chest pain, what doctors call *angina*. When the blood supply to the heart muscle is completely cut off, the heart muscle dies. This is called a heart attack or a *myocardial infarctio*n. In some cases, when there is a large amount of heart muscle damage, the remaining heart muscle is unable to pump blood to the rest of the body adequately. This is another cause of heart failure.

**Damage to the heart valves** A number of conditions, including heart attack, high blood pressure, bacterial infections of the valves (endocarditis), aging, and rheumatic fever, can damage the heart valves. As a result of this damage, the normal forward flow of blood through the heart is disrupted. This can sometimes result in a narrowing of the valve (called *stenosis*) or a leaking of the valve (called *insufficiency*).

When the valve becomes narrowed (*stenotic*), it causes an increased pressure within the heart. The heart has to push harder to get the same amount of blood out. Over years, this can damage the heart muscle and cause it to fail.

Other times, the valve can become leaky (or insufficient). This means that when the heart pushes the blood out, some of the blood pushed out comes back into the ventricle. This backward flow of blood is called *regurgitation* by doctors. When a valve is leaking like this, the heart has to pump harder and faster to keep the same amount of blood circulating. This can, over time, lead to heart muscle damage and eventual heart failure.

Severely damaged valves can either be fixed or replaced by surgeons.

**Cardiomyopathy** *Cardiomyopathy* is a disease of the heart muscle. The name comes from the roots *cardio* meaning "heart," *myo* meaning "muscle," and *pathy* meaning "disease." In cardiomyopathy, the heart muscle has been damaged and it does not work as efficiently as before. Cardiomyopathy can lead to an enlarged, poorly pumping heart.

In most people, the cause of cardiomyopathy is unknown. In some people, however, doctors are able to identify a cause or contributing factors, including some that affect the heart and cardiovascular system. For example, any of the following conditions may cause or contribute to cardiomyopathy:

- Sustained high blood pressure
- Heart tissue damage from a previous heart attack
- Chronic rapid heart rate
- Emphysema. Severe lung disease can result in **right-sided heart failure**.
- Nutritional deficiencies of essential vitamins and minerals, such as thiamin (vitamin B-1), selenium, calcium, and magnesium
- Low red-blood-cell count (severe anemia)
- Overactive or underactive thyroid gland (hyperthyroidism and hypothyroidism)
- Pregnancy. Heart failure may develop during the last 3 months of pregnancy or several months after pregnancy. The cause of this is not well understood, but it may be due to an abnormal immune system response.
- Excessive use of alcohol over many years
- Abuse of cocaine or antidepressant medications, such as tricyclic antidepressants
- Use of some chemotherapeutic drugs to treat cancer
- Certain viral infections, which may injure the heart and trigger cardiomyopathy

**Right-sided heart failure**

A malfunction of the right ventricle. An inability of the right ventricle to pump a sufficient amount of blood into the lungs.

- Hemochromatosis. This is a disorder in which your body doesn't properly metabolize iron, causing the accumulation of iron in your heart muscle.
- Arrhythmogenic right ventricular dysplasia (ARVD). This results in muscle tissue in the right ventricle being replaced by fat, triggering abnormal heart rhythms. In many people, there appears to be a genetic basis for ARVD.
- **Amyloidosis**. This is a disease that results from abnormal proteins or cell products being deposited in the heart muscle. The affected heart muscle is no longer able to pump blood.

**Amyloidosis**
This is a disorder in which insoluble protein fibers are deposited in tissues and organs (like the heart), impairing their function.

Fortunately, treating these conditions during their early stages can often prevent heart failure or significantly delay its onset. In order for a prevention strategy to work, the condition must be diagnosed early and an effective treatment strategy implemented. Treatment depends on what the cause of your heart failure is and what the condition of your heart is now. Medications, implantable devices, or in severe cases, a heart transplant are all possible treatments.

Victoria's comment:

*I developed heart failure when I was in my sixties. My doctor told me it developed because of long-term high blood pressure and coronary artery disease. I've been treated for both those conditions now and my heart failure has improved some.*

## 9. What is the difference between left-sided heart failure and right-sided heart failure?

It may be helpful to review the section in Question 7 that discusses the anatomy of the heart and how it works before reading this explanation.

When the left ventricle can't pump out enough blood, blood gets backed up in the lungs (behind the left ventricle), causing **pulmonary edema**. *Pulmonary edema* is a build-up of fluid in the lungs. This fluid in the lungs makes patients wheeze, cough, and become short of breath. This excess fluid or **congestion** explains the term *congestive heart failure*. As the heart's ability to pump decreases, blood flow slows down, causing fluid to build up in tissues throughout the body (**edema**). Edema is commonly noticed as swelling of the hands and feet. If it is prolonged, **left-sided heart failure** can eventually lead to right-sided heart failure.

The right atrium receives the "used" blood that returns to the heart through the veins; the right ventricle then pumps it into the lungs to be replenished with oxygen. When the right ventricle cannot pump out enough blood, it causes fluid to back up into the veins and capillaries of the body. Because of the back-up, fluid leaks out of the capillaries and builds up in the tissues, a condition called *systemic edema*. Edema is especially noticeable in the legs because gravity pulls the fluid into the lower half of the body.

Right-sided or right ventricular (RV) heart failure usually occurs as a result of left-sided failure. When the left ventricle fails, increased fluid pressure is transferred back through the lungs, ultimately damaging the heart's right side.

Victoria's comment:

*My heart failure is left-sided. The left side of my heart is enlarged and doesn't pump blood as effectively as before. I find that I get tired easily and that my legs swell up when I go off my diet or exercise too much.*

**Pulmonary edema**

Increased fluid in the lungs. This can result from heart failure and is a common cause of shortness of breath in CHF patients.

**Congestion**

An accumulation of excessive blood or fluid in the body's vessels or organs.

**Edema**

A swelling of the tissues of the body as a result of fluid overload.

**Left-sided heart failure**

A malfunctioning of the left ventricle that results in the backing up of fluid in the lungs.

**The Basics**

**Diastole**

Part of the normal cardiac cycle; the heart fills up with blood in preparation for ejecting it in the next phase of the cardiac cycle called systole.

**Systole**

That portion of the cardiac cycle in which the ventricles squeeze blood out of the heart.

**Systolic dysfunction**

An inability of the heart to squeeze enough blood out of the heart. It often results from dilation and scarring of the heart muscle.

**Diastolic dysfunction**

A malfunction of the left ventricle that occurs when the heart muscle enlarges and becomes too stiff. It becomes unable to stretch to receive enough blood and the heart output falls.

## 10. When discussing my heart failure, I've heard my doctor mention the terms "systolic" and "diastolic" dysfunction. What are they?

When your heart beats, it goes through two phases. In the first phase, the ventricles are at rest. The atria contract and pump blood into the ventricles; doctors call this phase **diastole** or the resting phase. In the second more active phase, called **systole**, the ventricles contract and force the blood out into the circulatory system.

Patients with heart failure have suffered from some condition that has damaged the heart muscle. The resulting damage weakens the ventricle (most often the left ventricle) so that it has difficulty pumping blood out to the rest of the body; this is known as **systolic dysfunction**.

In some cases of heart failure, the ventricle becomes stiff so that it has difficulty filling with blood; this is known as **diastolic dysfunction**. As a result, the amount of blood the heart can pump decreases, and the heart's ability to manage any additional workload is decreased.

It is important for your doctor to determine what type of dysfunction is causing your heart failure, because each type has different causes and different treatments.

## 11. What is the "ejection fraction"?

The **ejection fraction (EF)** is the measure of the percentage of blood that is ejected from the main pumping chamber of the heart (the left ventricle) with each beat. A heart does not pump all of the available blood out each time it beats. A normal heart pumps out or ejects only about 50 to 65 percent of the blood inside. If the heart is damaged, the ejection fraction frequently falls below 40 percent. However, you can have a normal ejection fraction and still have heart failure. This may be related to diastolic heart failure.

Although the ejection fraction is a useful number in some situations, it is not the whole story by any means. People with EFs of 40 percent can be severely disabled, while those with EFs of 15 percent may hardly have any symptoms at all.

Measuring the ejection fraction may be useful for the cardiologist following the course of the problem in some people.

Traditionally, the ejection fraction was measured by injecting the left ventricle with dye during a cardiac catheterization. After the injection, physicians watched the flow of the dye using an X-ray monitor. During this procedure, called a **ventriculogram**, physicians were able to measure the amount of dye that was pumped out of the left ventricle during a heartbeat. From this measure, the ejection fraction was established.

Today, the ejection fraction is mostly measured using sound waves during an **echocardiogram**. An echocardiogram is a safer and faster way of establishing the ejection fraction. Because an echocardiogram does not require the expertise, time, and special laboratory of a cardiac catheterization, ejection fractions can be measured frequently and can help doctors gauge the effectiveness of treatment.

**Ejection fraction (EF)**

The percentage of blood that is ejected from the left ventricle during each heartbeat. It is a measure of the effectiveness of the heart function.

*A normal heart pumps out or ejects only about 50 to 65 percent of the blood inside.*

**Ventriculogram**

A test that utilizes dye injected into the heart via a catheter. X-ray images are taken of the dye that outlines the inside of the heart. This allows cardiologists to observe the structure and function of the heart.

**Echocardiogram**

A test that employs sound waves to examine the anatomy and function of the heart.

The Basics

## 12. What type of doctor should I see for my heart failure?

Most people with heart failure are treated by either an internist or a cardiologist. Who you choose to be your treating physician depends on many factors. These factors might include:

- The doctor's training, board certification, and experience
- The proximity of the medical office to your home
- The doctor's participation in your insurance plan
- The doctor's reputation in the community
- Your ability to build a trusting relationship with the doctor
- The doctor's ability to speak your native language or understand your culture and customs

Although many of these issues do not necessarily bear on a doctor's clinical abilities, patients will often choose a doctor by what is most important to them.

It may be helpful to understand the difference between an internist and a cardiologist before you choose your physician. An *internist* is a man or woman who has attended 4 years of college, 4 years of medical school, and at least 3 years of a medical residency. During that residency, the internist studies the diagnosis and medical treatment of a wide variety of diseases of the human body, with emphasis on the heart, lungs, digestive tract, and the neurological (brain and nerves) and endocrine (e.g., thyroid, pancreas, and pituitary glands) systems. After completing the residency, the physician is invited by the American Board of Internal Medicine to take an examination to demonstrate his or her understanding of internal medicine. This is a grueling 2-day

examination, the successful completion of which enti-
tles the physician to be called board certified or a diplomate of the American Board of Internal Medicine.

The American Board of Internal Medicine created the
certification process to assure the public that a medical
specialist has successfully completed an approved edu-
cational program and an evaluation, including a secure
examination designed to assess the knowledge, experience, and skills requisite to the provision of high-
quality patient care.

Certification requirements include:

- Completion of a course of study leading to an M.D.
  or D.O. (doctor of osteopathy) degree from a recognized school of medicine or school of osteopathy
- Completion of required training in an accredited
  residency program
- Assessment and documentation of individual performance from the residency training director or
  from the chief of service in the hospital where the
  specialist practices
- An unrestricted license to practice medicine
- Passing a certification examination

A board-certified internist is capable of rendering excellent care to patients with congestive heart failure.

A *cardiologist* is a physician who has all the training of an
internist, including the 3-year residency, but then un-
dergoes an extra 3 to 4 years of training that focuses on
the heart. This training period is called a *cardiology fellowship*. The cardiologist spends years of in-depth study
learning about the diseases that affect the heart. After
successfully completing this fellowship, the cardiologist
is invited to sit for an examination by the American

Board of Internal Medicine in cardiologic diseases. If he or she passes the test, the cardiologist is referred to as being a board-certified cardiologist or a diplomate of the American Board of Internal Medicine, Cardiology. As a general rule, the cardiologist will have more training and experience in the area of heart failure.

There have been many studies comparing the care rendered to CHF patients by internists and cardiologists. In these studies, patients treated by cardiologists were significantly more likely to be admitted to an intensive care unit; receive chest X-rays, **electrocardiograms (EKGs or ECGs)**, nuclear medicine tests, cardiac catheterizations, and stress tests; and have their weight monitored daily than were patients treated by noncardiologists. This more intensive level of care rendered by cardiologists may result in improved symptoms and fewer visits to the hospital by the CHF patient. However, this more intensive management resulted in significantly greater costs than those of patients of generalists.

Interestingly, both cardiologists and internists did poorly when adhering to medication guidelines. The majority of patients with CHF who were eligible for an **ACE inhibitor**, a beta blocker, or an aldosterone antagonist did not receive these medications, regardless of the treating physician.

Victoria's comment:

*When I was first diagnosed with CHF, I was being treated by an internist. He was a good doctor, but told me that my condition was getting more serious and more complicated. My internist referred me to a cardiologist. I've been seeing my cardiologist for 8 years. I still see my internist for colds and my arthritis, but I see my cardiologist for my heart problems.*

**Electrocardiograms (EKGs or ECGs)**

Tests that measure the electrical waves in the heart.

**ACE inhibitor**

Angiotensin-converting-enzyme inhibitor; drug used to reduce elevated blood pressure, treat congestive heart failure, and alleviate strain on hearts damaged as a result of a heart attack. They work by stopping the body from making angiotensin, a substance in the blood that makes vessels tighten and raises blood pressure.

# PART TWO

# Diagnosis

How is CHF diagnosed?

What is an echocardiogram?

*More . . .*

*Heart failure is the common final pathway for many diseases.*

## 13. How is CHF diagnosed?

Heart failure is the common final pathway for many diseases, and so heart failure has many causes. The causes of heart failure range from malfunction of the heart valves to infections of the heart muscle to diseases of the bones and blood. It is not sufficient to say that a person has a diagnosis of heart failure without saying what the cause of the heart failure is, such as coronary artery disease or chronic hypertension. Therefore, a physician must investigate not only how the heart is malfunctioning, but why it is malfunctioning. The doctor arrives at this diagnosis based upon the findings of your medical history, physical examination, and a series of diagnostic tests.

## 14. How does a patient's medical history help to diagnose CHF?

Your doctor will ask you many questions about your symptoms and medical history. A frank discussion of your history and symptoms is very important in helping the doctor make an accurate diagnosis. Don't be afraid to "look bad" by admitting to a poor diet and absent exercise habits. In addition, don't downplay symptoms of chest pain, fatigue, and increasing shortness of breath.

A patient history gathers information about possible causes of heart failure including:

- History of heart murmurs
- Family history of cardiomyopathy
- Alcohol and illegal drug use (cocaine, heroin, anabolic steroids)
- Diet. For example, high-fat diets can lead to coronary artery disease or thiamine deficiency can lead to reversible cardiomyopathy.
- Medication history

- History of high blood pressure, including treatment
- History of childhood rheumatic fever
- History of endocarditis or intravenous drug use
- History of cancer treatment, especially some chemo-therapy and radiation treatments to the chest area
- Prior chest pains or heart attack
- Recent viral illness
- Recent pregnancy
- History of diabetes or amyloidosis

Victoria's comment:

*During my first visit to the cardiologist, I filled out many questionnaires about my health and my family's health. The cardiologist seemed to ask me questions for hours about what my symptoms were like, what I ate, how I cooked, what medications I was taking, and on and on. I see now that he was trying to find out what risk factors there were for my heart failure, but at the time it was a real pain in the neck.*

## 15. How does the physical examination help diagnose CHF?

During the examination, the physician looks for an underlying cause and assesses heart function. The doctor will listen closely to the patient's heart and lungs, examine the abdomen, and assess blood flow to the arms and legs. The doctor uses a stethoscope to detect abnormal heart sounds (also called *murmurs*) that may indicate a leaky or narrowed valve and to detect fluid accumulation in the lungs. The physician also looks for bulging (distended) veins in the neck, an enlarged liver, and for swelling (edema) in the arms, legs, and abdomen. These signs along with a history of heart disease strongly suggest heart failure.

Based upon the results of the exam, the doctor may order tests to further evaluate cardiac performance and determine the cause of any problems.

## 16. What do blood tests tell the physician?

Physicians use blood tests to evaluate the function of many organs in the body. Commonly ordered blood tests reveal the function of the kidneys, liver, and thyroid gland. Tests to measure serum cholesterol and triglyceride levels may help determine a risk for coronary artery disease. A count of the white blood cells under a microscope can help to reveal infections and a measure of red blood cells can reveal a critical decrease in red blood cells or anemia. *Anemia* is a blood condition that occurs either when there are not enough red blood cells or when there is not enough hemoglobin in the red blood cells. Hemoglobin is the iron-containing substance in red blood cells that enables the blood to transport oxygen through the body.

## 17. How does the B-type natriuretic peptide (BNP) blood test help to diagnose CHF?

BNP is a protein substance secreted from the heart ventricles in response to increases in blood pressure or dilation of the ventricles that occurs when heart failure worsens. BNP can be measured from a simple blood test. BNP blood levels increase when heart failure symptoms worsen and decrease when the heart failure condition is stable. The BNP level in a person with heart failure—even someone whose condition is stable—is higher than in a person with normal heart function. BNP can be used to distinguish causes of shortness of breath in CHF patients that may also have asthma, emphysema, or pneumonia.

Victoria's comment:

*After having CHF for 7 years, my doctor started ordering this blood test. I asked why he ordered a test to find out if I had CHF when he already knew that I had it. He says it helps him to tell if my medication is working well to control the CHF.*

## 18. How is a chest X-ray helpful?

A chest X-ray shows the size of your heart and whether there is fluid build-up around the heart in the lungs. It can also help to eliminate other causes of shortness of breath that can be confused with CHF, such as emphysema or pneumonia.

Victoria's comment:

*I've gotten an X-ray every time I go to the hospital with shortness of breath. It always shows that I have water in my lungs from my CHF. But I've heard of other patients who were treated for CHF when they had pneumonia, so I guess it's worth the effort.*

## 19. What does the electrocardiogram tell the doctor about CHF?

The EKG is a noninvasive test used to measure electrical activity in the heart. Electrical sensors, called leads, are attached to predetermined positions on the arms, legs, and the front part of your chest. These leads record electrical activity, heart rate, and heart rhythm. An EKG can diagnose abnormalities of the beating of the heart, called *arrhythmias* (see question 87 for more

*The EKG is a noninvasive test used to measure electrical activity in the heart.*

details), as well as enlargement of the heart muscle, called *hypertrophy*. An EKG can also help to diagnose a heart attack (a *myocardial infarction*), which is a common cause of heart failure.

Victoria's comment:

*I get an EKG about four times per year at my cardiologist's office and at least one more at my internist's office. I had a problem with coronary artery disease, so my doctors say they have to watch out for signs of heart attack. My cardiologist made a miniature copy of my EKG and I carry it in my purse in case I have trouble breathing and have to go to a doctor's office or an emergency room. It helps the doctors to see my old EKG when they are trying to decide if I have had any changes in the EKG that could indicate a heart attack.*

## 20. What is an echocardiogram?

An *echocardiogram*, referred to casually as a *cardiac echo* or just *echo*, is an ultrasound examination of the heart. It is a safe and painless test that can be completed in less than an hour. The echocardiogram employs sound waves to examine the heart's structure and motion. It can produce detailed images of the heart's chambers and valves. It is capable of measuring the size of the chambers to within small fractions of an inch as well as measuring the thickness of the walls of the heart. The echocardiogram can also measure the pressure change (or pressure gradient) between the left ventricle and the aorta. Doctors commonly use the echocardiogram to assess the pumping function of the heart by measuring the ejection fraction.

Normally, the heart ejects approximately 60 percent of the blood in the left ventricle every time the heart beats. Patients with ejection fractions of approximately

40–45 percent have mildly depressed ejection fractions; patients with ejection fractions of about 30–40 percent have moderately depressed ejection fractions; and patients with ejection fractions in the 10–25 percent range have severely depressed ejection fractions.

It is important to keep in mind that someone with a normal ejection fraction reading can still have heart failure. *Diastolic dysfunction* is a term physicians use to describe the effects of the heart muscle that has become so thick and stiff that the ventricle does not expand for blood coming in from the atrium. Therefore, the ventricle holds a smaller-than-usual volume of blood. While the percentage of blood pushed out in each heartbeat is high (the ejection fraction), the amount of blood pushed out in each heartbeat is low (the cardiac output). The patient suffers heart failure because the total amount of blood pumped isn't enough to meet the body's needs.

Victoria's comment:

*I mentioned before that I get an echocardiogram at least once a year from my cardiologist. He uses it to check my ejection fraction. I didn't know till I read this book that the echocardiogram can also look at the heart valves and aorta.*

## 21. What is a stress test?

In some cases, a cardiologist will use a less-invasive procedure called a *stress test* to assess the possibility of coronary heart disease. This test records the heart's activity during exercise, either walking on a treadmill or pedaling a stationary bike to see whether the heart responds normally to the stress of exercise. In other cases where the patient is incapable of this type of exercise, the cardiologist will infuse a drug into the bloodstream to increase the heart rate or to affect the flow of blood within the heart and an echocardiogram is used to obtain images of the heart. If the results of this procedure suggest the presence of coronary artery disease, a subsequent referral for cardiac catheterization is likely.

Victoria's comment:

*I had a stress test when I was first diagnosed with CHF. The doctors used a radioactive dye and a special camera to get an ejection fraction. The EKG on the stress test showed that I had some blockages in my coronary arteries. I eventually had them fixed with bypass surgery. The stress test is tiring and made me very short of breath.*

## 22. What is a cardiac catheterization?

A *cardiac catheterization* provides measurements of cardiac output and pressures within the heart and the major vessels going to and from the heart. During the test, a catheter (or hollow tube) is inserted through a large blood vessel and into the heart and is used to obtain these measurements. A dye is injected into the catheter that makes it easier to view the arteries and the structure of the heart by X-ray. A special camera is then used to determine how much of the dye is ejected from the heart with each beat. The infusion of dye typically produces a characteristic "hot flash" sensation throughout the body that lasts 10 to 15 seconds.

**Angina**

A medical term for chest pain that occurs because there is not enough oxygen in the heart.

Cardiologists perform catheterizations on patients with **angina** and in patients with a history of heart attack to determine if coronary artery disease is causing heart failure. This procedure produces X-ray images of the coronary arteries called *angiograms*, as well as images of the left ventricle. They are used to monitor heart function.

Major complications of angiography are rare (about 0.1 percent) but they can occur. They include stroke, heart attacks, and kidney damage. The more experienced the medical center in this procedure, the lower the risk.

## 23. What is a radionuclide ventriculography?

*Radionuclide ventriculography* is also called *multiple-gated acquisition scanning* or just *MUGA scan.* This nuclear medicine test involves injecting a small amount of radioactive dye into a vein, then taking pictures of the heart as it pumps blood. Technicians use a special camera to obtain images of the heart during rest and immediately following exercise on a treadmill. Like an echo, this test shows how much blood the heart can pump with each beat. The dye used for this test is typically iodine based. If you or any of your family members has ever had allergic reactions to shellfish (which contain iodine) or to iodine itself, be sure to tell the doctor before having this procedure.

The results of these tests also allow the doctor to determine the nature of the problem with the heart. The doctor uses this information, along with the ejection fraction reading, to determine what treatments would be most effective.

Victoria's comment:

*The radionuclide ventriculography was the type of heart scan that I had when I was first diagnosed. Now my cardiologist likes to use the echocardiogram to measure my ejection fraction. It's also a lot more convenient for me to go to his office rather than the hospital. Also, with the echocardiogram, I don't have to have an IV or get injected with dye.*

## 24. What is contrast-enhanced magnetic resonance imaging (MRI)?

A *magnetic resonance imaging (MRI) scan* is a technique used by radiologists and cardiologists to create a picture of the heart to see if it is working correctly. The scan does not use X-rays; rather, it uses powerful magnets and radio waves to create images of the heart. The images of the heart can be improved by using contrast agents to enhance the picture. Special contrast agents (also called *dyes*) are injected into the patient's arm while the MRI machine is taking a picture of the heart. When the contrast agent reaches the heart, it "lights up" the inside of the heart chambers. This makes it easier for doctors to see the structures inside of the heart. MRIs are helpful for identifying patients with irreversible heart damage. Damage appears as very bright areas on the scan.

# PART THREE

# *Exacerbations*

What is an "exacerbation" of CHF?

How do I know if my CHF
is getting worse?

What is a CHF action plan?

*More . . .*

## 25. What is an "exacerbation" of CHF?

An exacerbation of CHF is a sudden and prolonged worsening of a patient's CHF symptoms, such as an increased shortness of breath, mental confusion, leg swelling, fatigue, and weight gain. In severe cases, an exacerbation of CHF can be complicated by extreme shortness of breath. The patient even may report a feeling of drowning. The patient may cough up pink frothy sputum or may even become confused or unconscious. A CHF exacerbation is a medical emergency and requires the immediate attention of a doctor.

Exacerbations of CHF occur when there is an increased demand placed on the heart that the weakened heart cannot compensate for by beating harder or faster. These increased demands may be the result of cardiac or noncardiac changes. These exacerbations often are life threatening and can lead to hospitalization. The number of CHF exacerbations per year and the severity of exacerbations can increase as the disease progresses and the heart becomes less able to handle increased loads.

Heart failure exacerbations are very common reasons for hospitalization in the United States and Canada. In severe cases, the patient needs the mechanical support of a **ventilator** until the acute symptoms have resolved.

**Ventilator**

A machine that can push air into the lungs when a patient can no longer breathe for him- or herself.

In a study examining factors that lead to worsening CHF, nearly one third of incidents occurred because of patients' failure to comply with a medical regimen. For example, about 22 percent of patients did not restrict their intake of salt. Salt promotes the retention of water in the bloodstream, which can place an added strain on an already weakened heart. Eventually, excess water can back up into the lungs. Another 7 percent did not comply with instructions for taking their medication. In fact, many in this group stopped taking their medications altogether.

Some other causes of CHF exacerbation are:

- Excessive alcohol intake
- Lung infections
- Increased exercise
- Irregular heartbeats (both beats that are too fast and too slow)
- Coronary artery disease
- **Side effects** of medications (especially the use of negative inotropic drugs such as beta-blockers, disopyramide, verapamil, nifedipine, diltiazem)
- Increased high blood pressure
- Heart valve infections (endocarditis)
- Anemia

**Side effects**

Secondary reactions that result from a medication or therapy. Side effects of some heart failure medications include headache, nausea, dizziness, and low blood pressure.

Although this information may be frightening or even depressing, there is good news here. The most common causes of CHF exacerbation are within the control of the average patient. By attending to these factors, physicians and patients can help to prevent the commonest causes of CHF exacerbation. Managing these causes not only deals with the immediate decompensation, but also improves the prognosis for the future.

*The most common causes of CHF exacerbation are within the control of the average patient.*

Victoria's comment:

*In the first year after my diagnosis, I had several exacerbations of my CHF. I was hospitalized for each one. Eventually, I underwent a coronary artery bypass surgery and really watched how much I exercised and how much salt I cooked with. I haven't had an exacerbation in 3 years.*

## 26. How do I know if my CHF is getting worse?

Because early treatment of worsening CHF is most effective in preventing hospitalizations, it is very important for the patient to recognize when his symptoms are getting worse. The early symptoms or warning signs of a CHF exacerbation can be different for each person. The patient is the best person to know if he or she is having difficulty breathing, feeling more tired, or gaining more weight. Family members or friends may also recognize some of these signs. Therefore, it is important that you inform your family and friends of these warning signs and let them know what to do if they see them. A change or increase in the symptoms usually experienced may be the only early warning signs you get.

You may notice one or more of the following signs of worsening CHF:

- **Weight gain:** A gain of more than 3 pounds in 24 hours or 5 pounds in a week, no matter what your symptoms are.
- **Shortness of breath:** This symptom is called *dyspnea* by physicians; it can occur during activity, at rest, or while sleeping. It can come on gradually during the day or may come on suddenly and wake you from sleep. Patients with worsening CHF often have difficulty breathing while lying flat and may need to prop up the upper body and head on two pillows. They often complain of waking up tired or feeling anxious and restless. Shortness of breath occurs

**Pulmonary vein**

The large vein that leads from the lungs to the left atrium in the heart. It carries oxygenated blood to the left side of the heart.

when your blood "backs up" in the **pulmonary veins** (the vessels that return blood from the lungs to the heart) because the heart can't keep up with the supply. This causes fluid to leak into the lungs and it interferes with the lungs' ability to get oxygen into your body. Typically, the skin is clammy and pale; when severe, it can appear nearly blue. This is a life-threatening situation and the patient must go immediately to an emergency room (ER).

- **Persistent coughing or wheezing**: Though sometimes misinterpreted by patients and doctors as a chest cold or bronchitis, coughing and wheezing can be a sign of worsening CHF. It results from a build-up of fluid in the lungs. When it is severe, the patient may notice white or pink blood-tinged mucus. This is a serious sign and should prompt a call to your physician and requires a trip to the emergency room.

- **Swelling of the hands or feet**: A build-up of excess fluid in body tissues is a symptom called *edema* by physicians. It is a sign of worsening CHF. This excess fluid leads to swelling in the feet, ankles, legs, or abdomen or sometimes just weight gain. You may find that you can't get your rings on or that your shoes feel tight. As blood flow out of the heart slows, blood returning to the heart through the veins backs up, causing fluid to build up in the tissues. The kidneys are less able to dispose of **sodium** and water, also causing fluid retention in the tissues.

- **Excess tiredness**: If you're experiencing a tired feeling all the time or having difficulty with everyday activities, such as shopping, climbing stairs, carrying groceries, or walking, your CHF may be acting up. The fatigue happens because your heart can't pump enough blood to meet the needs of your body tissues. Your body then diverts blood away from less vital organs, particularly muscles in the limbs, and

**Sodium**

A mineral that works with potassium and calcium to control normal heart rhythm and water balance. A high-sodium diet can lead to high blood pressure in some people. In people who already have heart failure, too much sodium may make their condition worse.

sends it to the heart and brain. If this remains untreated, you may gradually lose muscle mass as the
tissues become oxygen depleted.

- **Appetite loss**: For some people, a loss of appetite or
  a feeling of being "stuffed" after eating a small meal
  can be a sign of worsening CHF. Others may experience nausea after eating. This occurs because the
  digestive system is receiving less blood, thus causing
  problems with digestion. The body shunts the blood
  away from the digestive system and to the brain and
  heart. Although appetites are often depressed, patients with congestive heart failure gain weight because they retain salt and water.

- **Confusion**: When CHF is severe, the heart has a
  hard time getting enough blood and oxygen to the
  brain. This can result in confusion, memory loss,
  and feelings of disorientation. The patient may
  have difficulty carrying on a conversation or reading a book. Other signs of poor circulation to the
  brain include prolonged headaches, forgetfulness,
  confusion, slurring of speech, and excessive sleepiness. A spouse or other caregiver may notice this
  before the patient does. This is why family members and caregivers should be made aware of these
  symptoms of worsening CHF. They should act
  quickly to call the physician or an ambulance when
  they see them.

- **Palpitations**: An increased heart rate or palpitations
  is a sign that your heart is working hard. It needs to
  work harder to make up for the loss in pumping capacity of the failing heart. Patients may complain of
  a racing heartbeat or throbbing in their chest.

- **Sleeping problems**: When the amount of fluid in
  the lungs increases, it becomes difficult to sleep. Patients with this condition often use more pillows to
  prop themselves up in bed, sleep in a chair instead of

a bed, or complain of waking up at night with shortness of breath.

- **Malaise**: Any feeling of ill health, increased fatigue,
  and lack of energy that continues for more than 24
  hours.
- **Cyanosis**: Any blue color in the lips or fingernails.

All patients with CHF should have an action plan to
deal with worsening symptoms. The action plan should
be developed with the help of your doctor and discussed with your family, friends, or caregivers.

Victoria's comment:

*I know that I'm getting into trouble when I can't lie down
in bed without getting short of breath. Through painful
experience and the nagging of my cardiologist, I have gotten into the habit of weighing myself every day. When my
weight increases more than a pound or two above the last
couple of days' weights, I know that I have to take more
diuretics and call my cardiologist. If I ignore it, I've found
that it doesn't take too long before I'm back in the emergency room.*

## 27. What is respiratory distress?

**Respiratory distress** is a medical term used to describe
severe shortness of breath. It occurs when there is not
enough oxygen in the blood due to problems with the
ability of the lungs to take in oxygen. When you are
in respiratory distress, you may be short of breath
and get out of breath by doing simple tasks such as
walking across a room, brushing your teeth, or sometimes just resting in a chair or in bed. Respiratory
distress occurs in CHF patients when the fluid backs
up in the lungs (called *pulmonary edema*). Respiratory

*Respiratory
distress is a
medical term
used to
describe severe
shortness of
breath.*

**Exacerbations**

**Respiratory
distress**

A difficulty in
breathing; shortness
of breath at rest.

distress is a serious condition that should prompt patients to call their doctor or an ambulance. Respiratory distress can lead to **respiratory failure**.

Victoria's comment:

*I've been in respiratory distress several times. It's an experience I try hard not to repeat. At first it feels like you have a cold or bronchitis. Then the wheezing and shortness of breath get worse. For me it took almost a week to get really bad. Then, I felt like I couldn't catch my breath or I was drowning. My husband had to call an ambulance to get me to the emergency room. I spent a week in the hospital.*

## 28. What is respiratory failure?

*Respiratory failure* is a life-threatening situation in which the respiratory system stops functioning properly. Respiratory failure occurs when the lungs and respiratory system become unable to provide the body with sufficient oxygen and fail to "blow off" accumulated carbon dioxide. If the major cause of respiratory failure is an inability of the lungs to get in enough oxygen to meet the body's oxygen requirement, then it is referred to as *hypoxemic respiratory failure.*

Respiratory failure in CHF can be very gradual and may progress slowly over hours or days. Acute respiratory failure is characterized by the onset of shortness of breath that occurs over hours or days. This can occur in CHF patients when they exercise too much, don't take their medicines, or have too much salt in their diets. It can also occur when the patient acquires a lung infection or is exposed to lung irritants that cause inflammation and increased mucous production.

**Respiratory failure**

A decreased ability to get enough oxygen or inability to breathe at all, it results in a decrease in oxygen in the blood and increased carbon dioxide in the blood.

CHF can lead to severe respiratory failure. In respiratory failure, there can come a point where the failure becomes so marked that the body becomes deprived of oxygen or the level of carbon dioxide too high. When these conditions occur, other organs can begin to fail as well from the lack of oxygen. The brain is particularly sensitive to lack of oxygen and the build-up of carbon dioxide. In this state, the patient can become confused, unable to make appropriate decisions about his or her treatment, may lose consciousness, go into a coma, and if this state is prolonged and the oxygen levels become too low, the patient can die.

Clearly, severe respiratory failure is a medical emergency; the patient is critically ill and requires the attention of a physician and needs to be admitted to the hospital. Because of the effect of respiratory failure on the brain, it is inappropriate to allow the patient in severe failure to make decisions about visiting the doctor or emergency room. This is a situation in which a relative or friend must make decisions for the patient and get the proper emergency care.

## 29. If I'm having trouble breathing, do I need to wait for my doctor to return my call or can I start treatment myself?

Severe respiratory symptoms are a life-threatening emergency. Early aggressive treatment is recommended by experts. You are the one who can first tell if you're starting to get short of breath. Therefore, you are the one who can react most quickly to this warning sign.

Dealing with occasional worsening symptoms is part of living with CHF. You should discuss with your doctor what to do when this happens, so you're prepared to deal with it quickly. Based on your history and physical condition, your doctor may recommend that you call the ambulance to be evaluated in the emergency room of the local hospital, or the doctor may recommend a more conservative approach of self-treatment and reevaluation. You should discuss with your doctor what medications you should take when you first start to get short of breath.

A written list of medications that includes how much to take and when to take them should be approved by your doctor and stored in an easily accessible place. This list and these medications should be part of every CHF patient's "action plan" for treatment of exacerbations. You should always have a supply of all necessary medications handy so you don't have to wait to get them from a pharmacy in an emergency.

Victoria's comment:

*I've found that waiting to see if you get better is never a good option. I usually get worse if I ignore my symptoms. Now, if I feel myself getting short of breath or I see that my weight has increased, I call my cardiologist. He asks a lot of questions about fever and cough, as well as chest pain, palpitations, or fainting. If I say no to these questions, he often tells me to rest and increase my diuretic, and he calls me back in a few hours to make sure that I'm getting better.*

*Every CHF patient should have an action plan for getting emergency care quickly in the event of severe symptoms.*

## 30. What is a CHF action plan?

Every CHF patient should have an action plan for getting emergency care quickly in the event of severe symptoms. The action plan should consist of the following.

### Things you'll need at home:

- Contact information for doctor, hospital, therapists, pharmacists, ambulance, and friends or family who can help in an emergency. This information should be prominently displayed near the telephone.
- Written directions to the doctor's office, clinic, or hospital. You may not be able to talk easily, so giving directions will be difficult.
- Written information on when to call the doctor, under what circumstances, and how frequently
- A schedule of medications and what dosages to take under specific circumstances
- A copy of your last EKG
- An accurate bathroom scale
- Know what your normal "dry" weight is and your current weight is. Your "dry weight" is your weight when you've been taking your diuretics and you have no shortness of breath and no hand swelling
- A list of those signs or symptoms that should prompt an immediate visit to the doctor's office
- A list of those signs or symptoms that should prompt an immediate call for an ambulance and a visit to the ER

### Things you'll need if you go to the doctor's office or hospital:

- A complete list of your medications and dosages (prescription and over-the-counter), vitamins, and inoculations, and the prescribing doctor
- A list of any over-the-counter (OTC) medications, cold remedies, herbal cures, homeopathic treatments, teas, or cultural-based treatments such as acupuncture, cupping, or coin rolling that you are currently undergoing

- All medications or other substances to which you have known allergic reactions
- If you have them, you should bring copies of your most recent EKG or similar tests/reports
- What your normal "dry" weight is and what your current weight is
- Some cash to spend
- An updated copy of your advance directive, **medical proxy**, or medical **power of attorney** form and organ donation card if applicable
- A description of your medical history, in chronological sequence (including your use of tobacco, alcohol, or drugs)
- Insurance company cards or at least names and policy numbers
- Names, addresses, and phone numbers of your next-of-kin

This action plan should be developed with the help of your physician, after a full assessment of the following:

- Availability and response times of ambulances
- Availability of friends and family who can drive in an emergency
- Proximity to an ER or doctor's office
- Availability of relatives or friends who can stay with the patient until the patient improves or a visit to the doctor is decided on

After this assessment, you can develop an action plan with your doctor and determine the appropriate treatment steps for signs and symptoms of respiratory difficulty, chest pain, or increased leg swelling. Family members and those that are close to you should be informed and participate in this emergency action plan.

**Medical proxy**

An advance directive whereby a patient gives decision-making power about his or her health care to another in case he or she is unable to communicate for themselves.

**Power of attorney**

An advance directive. This is legal permission for another adult to act on your behalf, epecially in legal or health matters.

Victoria's comment:

*I've gone over most of these issues with my cardiologist. I have a copy of my EKG that I carry in my purse. My husband knows what to do when I start getting short of breath, and I've written the numbers of my doctors and local ambulance by the phone so I can get them in an emergency. I think these are important things to do and they have been helpful to me more than once.*

## 31. Are there things I shouldn't do when my CHF gets worse?

Although there are many effective measures to treat signs and symptoms of CHF while you're at home, there are also actions that should be avoided. Doing any of the following could make your condition worse:

- Do not take any extra doses of any medication that you have not discussed first with your doctor as part of your emergency action plan.
- Do not avoid taking your regular medicine in favor of taking unapproved medicines, alternative medicines, or home remedies.
- Do not take any substance that may suppress your breathing. Things that can suppress your breathing and that should be avoided include:
  - Alcohol
  - Codeine or other cough suppressants
  - Prescription pain killers, especially morphine and its derivatives
  - Sedatives, sleeping pills, or other sleep aids
- Do not engage in any exercise, even walking short distances, cooking, or cleaning. This will make your condition worse.
- Do not travel anywhere that makes it more difficult for you to speak to your doctor or get to a hospital.

## 32. How is a CHF exacerbation treated?

How the doctor treats your CHF exacerbation depends on how severe it is. You may have to visit your doctor's office or go to an outpatient clinic, or it may even require you to be admitted to the hospital for treatment.

Initially, the head of the patient's bed should be elevated. This reduces the amount of blood returning to the heart and makes it easier for the heart to pump. Patients may be most comfortable in a sitting position with their legs dangling over the side of the bed. The patient should eliminate any factors that may have contributed to the exacerbation when possible, such as resting if they've been too active or taking medication they may have forgotten to take. They should restrict fluid and salt.

The doctor should treat low blood cell counts (also known as anemia) as well as low thyroid hormone levels (called hypothyroidism) if they are present.

Doctors usually use a combination of medications when treating CHF exacerbations. Therapy generally starts with **nitrates** and **diuretics** if the patient's blood pressure and pulse are stable. The following are some of the medications that may be used during an acute exacerbation of CHF.

- **Diuretics** or "water pills" such as furosemide and hydrochlorothiazide help your kidneys to get rid of excess salt and water. They can be given by mouth or intravenously and work quickly.
- **Vasodilators** are a class of medications that include **nitroglycerin**. As their name implies, they dilate the

**Nitrates**

A medication that results in the dilation of blood vessels and a decrease in blood pressure, making it easier for blood to flow. They are used to treat chest pain and heart failure. Nitroglycerin tablets are examples.

**Diuretics**

Also known as a **water pill**; a medication that increases the excretion of water and salt from the body. It helps the kidneys eliminate salt and water from the bloodstream and increases the rate of urine formation. This helps to reduce high levels of fluid in people with heart failure.

**Vasodilators**

Medication that widens or relaxes the walls of blood vessels. ACE inhibitors, angiotensin II receptor blockers, nitroglycerin, and calcium channel blockers are vasodilators.

blood vessels and decrease the pressure on your heart, making it easier to pump blood.

- **Inotropes** are medications that increase the contractility of the heart and make it pump more effectively. This class of drugs includes the drug dobutamine.
- **Natriuretic peptides**. Nesiritide (brand name Natrecor) is a new drug for the treatment of CHF. In fact, it has emerged as one of the first new treatments for acute CHF in more than a decade. The body produces these proteins that appear to have an effect on easing the heart's workload when it's unable to pump blood efficiently. The new natriuretic peptide–based treatments are alternatives to inotropes and vasodilators.
- **Oxygen** In order to increase the amount of oxygen in your blood, the doctor may provide a higher concentration of oxygen in the air you breathe. Oxygen can be delivered by nasal prongs or by a face mask. The added oxygen may help reduce shortness of breath and make your heart beat more effectively.

If you are having severe difficulty breathing on your own and are not responding to medication, your lungs may need help in getting oxygen in the blood. Some ways of increasing the level of oxygen in your blood include using continuous positive airway pressure, **endotracheal intubation**, and a mechanical ventilator.

## 33. What is CPAP?

Continuous positive airway pressure (CPAP) and bi-level positive airway pressure (BiPAP) are methods of increasing the amount of oxygen a patient breathes. A face mask is placed securely over the patient's nose and mouth and a mechanical ventilator forces air into the patient's lungs. Recently, a study comparing nasal CPAP therapy and face mask ventilation therapy demonstrated

**Exacerbations**

**Nitroglycerin**

A type of nitrate medication, it dilates blood vessels. **Nitroglycerin (intravenous)** is the IV form of nitroglycerin and is a fast-acting vasodilator that is often given in the hospital to treat severe heart failure.

**Inotropes**

Drugs that stimulate the heart to contract more forcefully. IV inotropes are given to treat severe heart failure and include dobutamine, milrinone, and dopamine.

**Endotracheal intubation**

This is a procedure by which a tube is inserted through the mouth down into the trachea (the large airway from the mouth to the lungs). It is used to help connect a patient to a ventilator.

decreased need for intubation rates when these modalities are used. CPAP and BiPAP cannot be used in confused, uncooperative, combative, or unconscious patients. CPAP is easier and less invasive to use than putting an endotracheal tube in the patient's throat.

## 34. What is endotracheal intubation?

*Endotracheal intubation* utilizes a plastic flexible tube that is placed in the patient's windpipe. The tube is connected to the ventilator and oxygen is forced into the patient's lungs. Endotracheal intubation is an effective way to treat patients who are confused or unconscious. Unconscious patients are at risk for vomiting and then inhaling the vomitus into their lungs. This can result in a serious and sometimes fatal pneumonia called *aspiration pneumonia*. Endotracheal intubation can help to prevent this complication.

## 35. What is a ventilator?

The *ventilator* is a machine designed to provide artificial respiration for a patient with respiratory failure of any cause. The ventilator pumps humidified air (with a measured amount of oxygen) into the lungs via the endotracheal tube or tracheostomy tube. The elasticity of the lungs allows the expulsion of the air. Doctors use ventilators to control the amount of oxygen in the blood and the volume of air flowing into the lungs. In the hospital, ventilators are carefully monitored and adjusted only by people who are qualified to do so. These include respiratory therapists, nurses, and doctors.

Ventilators are very effective in treating respiratory failure, but they are not without their own problems. For example, ventilators may interfere with the ability to communicate and swallow. Ventilators can increase the blood levels of oxygen and decrease carbon dioxide levels, but they don't reverse the underlying disease. Patients complain that it is very unnatural to have a machine breathe for them and the endotracheal tubes can be uncomfortable. Therefore, many patients need to get extra sedation while on the ventilator. Finally, while on the ventilator, physicians need to take many blood tests and X-rays to monitor the disease progress and efficiency and safety of the ventilator.

*Avoid using salt in your cooking.*

Exacerbations

## 36. How do I prevent CHF exacerbations?

In many studies of CHF patients who come to the emergency department, one very common cause of CHF exacerbation was the failure to restrict salt in the diet. You should discuss this issue with your doctor or dietitian. Learn how to read food packages for their salt content. Avoid using salt in your cooking. Don't eat high-salt foods when you are out to eat.

Another common cause of CHF exacerbations is non-compliance with medication regimen. There are many reasons for which a patient will stop taking medications. Some experience unpleasant side effects; some cannot afford to buy the medication; others forget or don't want to accept the fact that they are sick and need the medication. Medications given for CHF are not optional; they are a necessary, lifesaving part of your daily schedule. If you have a problem with a medication, discuss it with your doctor. Many drug side effects decrease or disappear after a few weeks. Some don't go away, but by changing the drug to another brand or different class, your doctor can achieve the same beneficial effects while avoiding the unpleasant side effects.

If the drugs prescribed to you are too expensive, there may be ways to get them cheaper or even for free. Your doctor may be able to switch your medications to ones that are covered by your insurance plan or change them to a cheaper, but equally effective generic drug. The doctor may have drug samples for you to supplement the drugs you have to buy. Failing that, the drug companies themselves have programs for distributing medications free of charge for patients who cannot afford them. Patients should discuss the issue of drug affordability with their physicians and a social worker. A lot can be done to help you get your medications. Seeking help is a much better plan than stopping the medications.

Coronary artery disease is a common cause of CHF. Some ways to help prevent coronary artery disease include using small amounts of alcohol and quitting smoking. The intake of small amounts of alcohol, especially red wine, is sometimes recommended for the prevention of coronary artery disease. However, alcohol taken in larger amounts can interfere with the heart's ability to pump blood. Specifically, it can depress the contractility of the heart muscle and can cause irregular heartbeats. Alcohol can also cause cardiomyopathy and high blood pressure. Complete abstinence from alcohol is crucial for patients with alcohol-induced cardiomyopathy. Generally, patients with CHF should use alcohol sparingly (one glass or less per day) and only after a discussion with their cardiologist. Smoking decreases the amount of oxygen your heart gets, and the nicotine in tobacco causes your blood vessels to constrict and makes your heart work harder. Patients with CHF should stop smoking. If you cannot stop smoking by yourself, speak to your doctor about a smoking cessation plan.

Lung infections can result in less oxygen getting to the heart. To help prevent lung infections, patients with CHF should receive influenza vaccine yearly and a pneumococcal vaccination every 5 years. These can prevent some lung infections and reduce the amount of CHF exacerbations.

Attention to a patient's other medical problems is of major importance when considering how to decrease CHF exacerbations. Weight loss for obese patients, cessation of tobacco use, diagnosis and treatment of anemia, and an aggressive treatment of high cholesterol and triglycerides as well as tight control of blood sugar in diabetics must be stressed.

Mild exercise performed regularly may improve exercise capacity and decrease symptoms. For people with severe disease, exercise may be safer in a supervised environment surrounded by physicians and nurses. Investigation of local cardiac rehabilitation programs may be fruitful.

Victoria's comment:

*My doctor regularly goes over these issues with me. He especially is concerned about my salt intake and my weight. This is a struggle for me and while I've made improvements in both areas, I still have room for improvement. My cardiologist always asks me to bring my medications with me and he asks about each medication while I'm in the office. Sometimes he changes the medications if I'm having a problem or a side effect. One of my blood pressure medications made me cough all the time. He changed it to another medication in the same category and I didn't have that problem again. I told him that the diuretics keep me going to the bathroom all night. He suggested that I take them in the morning, so at night I wouldn't be awakened so often. That suggestion helped too. My point is talking with my doctor about my medications has made it easier for me to take them—even when I just wanted to throw them out the window.*

## 37. How do I make sure I'm treated according to my wishes if I can't speak?

In the past, if you were so sick that you were unable to communicate your wishes, the physician or the physician and family members made choices about how to care for you. Now, most physicians and hospitals ask patients to think about these issues while they are well and make them known in a formalized document.

Victoria's comment:

*This just seemed to make sense to me. My doctor asked me during a regular visit if I wanted to make some decisions now about how I'll be treated if I can't make decisions for myself. I talked to him about what I wanted done and what I didn't want done. I signed a form in his office to that effect. I went home and discussed it with my husband and had him fill out a form about his wishes. My doctor has a copy of this form and I have a copy that I keep with my copy of my EKG. Just in case.*

The following instruments are formalized ways to assure that you are treated according to your wishes:

**Advance directive** An *advance directive* is a general term that refers to your oral and written instructions about your future medical care, in the event that you become unable to speak for yourself. Each state regulates the use of advance directives differently. There are two types of advance directives: a **living will** and a medical power of attorney.

**Living will** A *living will* is a type of advance directive in which you put in writing your wishes about medical treatment should you be unable to communicate at the end of life. Your state law may define when the living

---

Advance
directive *is a
general term
that refers to
your oral and
written
instructions
about your
future medical
care, in the
event that you
become unable
to speak for
yourself.*

**Advance
directive**

This tells your doctor
what kind of care
you would like to
have if you become
unable to make
medical decisions.

**Living will**

An advance direc-
tive; it tells health
care workers about
your wishes if
you are unable to
communicate.

will goes into effect and may limit the treatments to which the living will applies. Your right to accept or refuse treatment is protected by constitutional and common law.

**Medical power of attorney** A *medical power of attorney* (also known as a durable power of attorney for health care, an appointment of a health care agent, or a health care proxy) is a document that enables you to appoint someone you trust to make decisions about your medical care if you cannot make those decisions yourself. The person you appoint may be called your health care agent, surrogate, attorney-in-fact, or proxy. In many states, the person you appoint through a medical power of attorney is authorized to speak for you at any time you are unable to make your own medical decisions, not only at the end of life.

**Do not resuscitate (DNR) order** A **do not resuscitate order** is another kind of advance directive. A DNR is a request not to have cardiopulmonary resuscitation (CPR) if your heart stops or if you stop breathing. You can use an advance directive form or tell your doctor that you don't want to be resuscitated. In this case, a DNR order is put in your medical chart by your doctor. DNR orders are accepted by doctors and hospitals in all states.

Most patients who die in a hospital have had a DNR order written for them. Patients who are not likely to benefit from CPR include people who have cancer that has spread, people whose kidneys don't work well, people who need a lot of help with daily activities, or people who have severe infections such as pneumonia that require hospitalization. If you already have one or more of these conditions, you should discuss your wishes about CPR with your doctor, either in the doctor's office or when you go to the hospital. It's best to do this early,

**Medical proxy**

An advance directive whereby a patient gives decision-making power about his or her health care to another in case he or she is unable to communicate.

**Do not resuscitate (DNR) order**

This is a type of advance directive. A DNR is a request not to have cardiopulmonary resuscitation if your heart stops or if you stop breathing.

before you are very sick and are considered unable to make your own decisions.

## 38. Why should I have an advance directive?

Every patient should have an advance directive. It gives you a voice in decisions about your medical care when you are unconscious or too ill to communicate. As long as you are able to express your own decisions, your advance directive will not be used and you can accept or refuse any medical treatment you like. Nevertheless, if you become seriously ill, you may lose the ability to participate in decisions about your own treatment.

Helen's comment:

*When my husband was dying of cancer, he became very short of breath. The doctors didn't want to him on a mechanical ventilator, but because there was no advance directive order in his medical chart, his doctor asked me to sign a DNR order. I sat there and thought about it for as long as I could. My husband had not been conscious for a week and was in tremendous pain. Though he had been sick for more than a year, we never wanted to discuss this type of situation. I sat there, looking at him. He was perspiring and gasping for air. I couldn't see that putting him on a ventilator would help him, but I didn't want him to die. I eventually signed the DNR order and the doctors gave him morphine to make him more comfortable. He died later that night. That was the most painful, agonizing decision I ever made. It is imperative that we appoint a health care agent or someone, maybe a family member, with the authority to speak for us when are unable to make our own medical decisions at any time of illness. We should tell them what we want to happen in this situation.*

*It is unfair and a painful burden for them to have to make the decision for you.*

# PART FOUR

# Treatment

What are the usual medications that
doctors prescribe for CHF patients?


Are pacemakers used to treat
heart failure?


Is alternative or complementary
medicine helpful in CHF?


*More . . .*

## NONSURGICAL TREATMENT

### *39. What are the usual medications that doctors prescribe for CHF patients?*

Physicians use various types of medications when treating patients with CHF, each of which has a different function. Although the symptoms of CHF can be treated and improved by therapy, your doctor will also want to diagnose and treat the underlying cause of CHF in an attempt to prevent progression and worsening of symptoms.

A study of conventional medications for the treatment of CHF reported the following percentages of use:

- Diuretics, 82%
- ACE inhibitors, 53%
- Nitrates, 49%
- Digitalis, 46%
- **Potassium**, 40%
- Aspirin, 36%
- **Calcium channel blockers**, 20%
- Coumadin (Warfarin), 17%
- Beta blockers, 15%
- Magnesium, 10%

**Note:** It is important to remember when being treated for heart failure that you should not take other medicines unless they have been discussed with your doctor. This especially includes OTC (nonprescription) medicines for appetite control, asthma, colds, cough, hay fever, or sinus problems, since they may tend to increase your blood pressure.

Helen's comment:

*To get the best results from your medications, you must take the drugs as directed.*

**Potassium**

A mineral that works with sodium and calcium to help control normal heart rhythm and water balance. Potassium also helps with normal muscle function.

**Calcium channel blockers (CCBs)**

Drugs that lower blood pressure by relaxing arteries and veins.

*During a recent illness I was not consistent in following my medicine schedule, sometimes forgetting and sometimes deliberately refusing to take my medicine. As a result, I suffered a relapse and was rushed to the ER of a local hospital.*

*Needless to say, I really learned the importance of taking my medicine "as prescribed".*

## 40. What are diuretics?

*Diuretics* are medications that cause the kidney to excrete more water and salt. Diuretics can cause the depletion of potassium and magnesium, which can be dangerous. Patients who are taking diuretics, therefore, should consult with their physician regarding supplementation of these electrolytes.

Also called *water pills*, diuretics are used to treat conditions such as CHF, high blood pressure (hypertension), or edema (water retention). Diuretics are also effective for the treatment of certain kinds of kidney or liver diseases.

Diuretics come in three basic types: the thiazides, the loop diuretics, and the potassium-sparing diuretics.

*Thiazide diuretics* work by increasing the excretion of water and salt from the kidneys. They are the only type of diuretic that dilates the blood vessels, which also helps to lower blood pressure. Some examples of thiazide diuretics are:

| Generic Name | Brand Name |
|---|---|
| methyclothiazide | Aquatensen |
| hydrochlorothiazide | Hydrodiuril |
| chlorthalidone | Hygroton |
| metolazone | Zaroxolyn |

*Diuretics are medications that cause the kidney to excrete more water and salt.*

Treatment

*Loop diuretics* cause the kidneys to increase the flow of urine. This helps reduce the amount of water in your body and lower your blood pressure. Common examples of loop diuretics are:

| **Generic Name** | **Brand Name** |
| --- | --- |
| furosemide | Lasix and Myrosemide |
| bumetanide | Bumex |
| torsemide | Demadex |
| ethacrynic acid | Edecrin |

*Potassium-sparing diuretics* are used to reduce the amount of water and salt in the body. Although these diuretics cause the body to lose a type of salt called sodium (table salt), they do not cause your body to lose another type of salt called potassium. Potassium levels should be checked frequently when beginning this type of diuretic, because high potassium levels can result, which are dangerous.

Some examples of potassium-sparing diuretics are:

| **Generic Name** | **Brand Name** |
| --- | --- |
| spironolactone | Aldactone |
| triamterene | Dyrenium |
| amiloride | Midamor |

## 41. What are the side effects of diuretics?

*Side effects* are unwanted conditions caused by a drug. These might include, for example, getting a rash from taking penicillin or a headache from taking nitroglycerin. Diuretics can cause side effects and patients should be aware of them and notify their doctor if they experience them. Common side effects of diuretics are:

- Weakness
- Muscle cramps
- Skin rash
- Increased sensitivity to sunlight (especially with thiazide diuretics)
- Vomiting
- Diarrhea
- Cramps
- Dizziness or lightheadedness
- Joint pain
- Palpitations

## 42. What are ACE inhibitors?

ACE inhibitors and vasodilators expand blood vessels, thereby allowing the heart to function more efficiently. Before discussing what ACE inhibitors are, it is appropriate to discuss what ACE is.

ACE stands for **a**ngiotensin-**c**onverting **e**nzyme. As you could assume from its name, ACE is an enzyme in the blood that converts a protein called *angiotensin* into an active form. Activated angiotensin causes the blood vessels in the body to constrict, which raises the blood pressure. Angiotensin also causes the body to release aldosterone, a substance that causes our kidneys to retain sodium and fluid, causing edema. By blocking the conversion of angiotensin to its active form, ACE inhibitors decrease blood pressure.

ACE inhibitors have been found to decrease or prevent the changes in the heart muscle that occur after heart muscle injury such as a heart attack. Some patients, especially those who develop heart muscle damage in the anterior wall of the heart, develop late swelling or dilation (called *heart remodeling* by cardiologists) in the left ventricle. This dilation significantly increases morbidity and reduces survival rate. Treating these patients early with ACE inhibitors has been demonstrated to slow the progression of left ventricular enlargement and reduce morbidity and mortality. When treated with ACE inhibitors, patients experience less heart dilation. A number of large-scale clinical trials have been completed that document the efficacy of such intervention.

ACE inhibitors are also prescribed for certain kinds of kidney problems, especially if you have diabetes.

Examples of common ACE inhibitors:

| Generic Name | Brand Name |
| --- | --- |
| benazepril | Lotensin |
| captopril | Capoten |
| enalapril | Vasotec |
| fosinopril | Monopril |
| lisinopril | Prinivil |
| quinapril | Accupril |

## 43. What are some side effects of ACE inhibitors?

About 10 percent of heart failure patients develop a chronic, irritating cough from ACE inhibitor use. This cough may resolve on its own, but if not, other brands of ACE inhibitors or newer drugs called ARBs can be used (see the following question). Other, less common side effects of ACE inhibitors are:

- Swelling of the lips, tongue, or throat (called *angioedema*)
- Diarrhea
- Headache

- Loss of taste or a taste of stainless steel in your mouth
- Loss of appetite
- Upset stomach
- Skin that is sensitive to sunlight
- Tired feeling
- Dizziness, lightheadedness, or fainting

If you experience any of these side effects, call your doctor. Do not stop the medication on your own. If you stop taking your medicine without checking with your doctor, it can worsen your condition.

## 44. I've heard the term ARBs when talking about medicine for CHF. What are ARBs?

ARB stands for **angiotensin receptor blocker**. It is a drug, like the ACE inhibitors (see the previous question), that blocks the effects of angiotensin on the body. In other words, ARBs reduce blood pressure by dilating blood vessels, decrease the body's ability to absorb salt and water by preventing the excretion of aldosterone, and decrease dilation of the heart muscle after heart attacks. Patients who are unable to take ACE inhibitors because of a severe cough should be considered for treatment with ARBs. Unlike ACE inhibitors, ARBs do not cause coughing, are well tolerated by patients, and cause no known class-specific side effects.

Currently, national consensus guidelines recommend that ARBs should be reserved for hypertensive patients who cannot tolerate ACE inhibitors (ACEIs). ARBs, however, are moving to the forefront of therapy with a promising role in the area of CHF treatment. In fact, a study called the Valsartan Heart Failure

*Angiotensin II receptor blockers (ARBs)*

Medications that lower blood pressure similarly to ACE inhibitors. ARBs are different because they stop angiotensin from working (instead of stopping the body from making them).

*Nitrates are a class of drug that causes dilation of the blood vessels in the body.*

Trial, published in 2001, adds to the growing body of evidence that ARBs may decrease symptoms of shortness of breath and swelling as well as reducing the mortality rate in CHF patients.

Some examples of ARBs:

| Generic Name | Brand Name |
|---|---|
| candesartan | Cilexetil |
| eprosartan | Teveten |
| irbesartan | Avapro |
| losartan | Cozaar |
| valsartan | Diovan |

## 45. What are nitrates and how are they used in CHF patients?

Nitrates are a class of drug that causes dilation of the blood vessels in the body. The dilation of blood vessels reduces the blood pressure and the amount of work the heart has to do to circulate blood. Nitroglycerin was used in the management of chest pain as early as 1879. Now, nitrates can be given to CHF patients to reduce symptoms. Nitrates can be administered in many forms, including sublingual, oral, topical, and intravenously.

When given chronically, nitrate therapy in CHF improves a patient's exercise tolerance. In combination therapy with other blood vessel dilators such as hydralazine, nitrates reduce mortality, although to a lesser extent than the ACE inhibitor enalapril.

When treating pulmonary edema, intravenous or sublingual nitrates are first-line agents. When CHF is severe and not responding to standard medical therapy, a short course of intravenous nitroglycerin can help break the vicious spiral of CHF.

Giving nitrates continually can result in their being less effective. Because this tolerance occurs, doctors recommend a nightly nitrate-free interval when prescribing nitrates for CHF in order to maintain maximal benefit during the hours of activity. The dosing can be increased later as necessary.

Common examples of nitrate medications are:

| Generic Name | Brand Name |
| --- | --- |
| nitroglycerin | Nitro-Dur, Nitrostat |
| isosorbide dinitrate | IMDUR, Isordil |
| isosorbide mononitrate | ISMO, Monoket |

Side effects from nitrates are few, regardless of the route of administration. The most common adverse effects are:

- Low blood pressure (hypotension)
- Headache
- Nausea
- Slow heartbeat (**bradycardia**)
- Skin reactions (caused by topical nitrates)

*Bradycardia*
A slow heartbeat.

## 46. What is hydralazine?

Hydralazine widens blood vessels, easing blood flow and increasing circulation. It also may increase the contractility of the heart muscle. Hydralazine is not as frequently used as diuretics and ACE inhibitors, but does have a place in CHF therapy. Hydralazine is often combined with other medications, such as nitrates, to reduce CHF symptoms. Physicians have found that hydralazine therapy increases resting cardiac performance as well as increasing the patient's ability to exercise. There is also evidence that improved cardiac performance is sustained at least in some patients during maintenance hydralazine therapy.

It is not known if using hydralazine on all CHF patients results in decreased mortality. Nevertheless, some studies suggest that in patients with severe chronic CHF, and in African-Americans, hydralazine therapy provides a better prognosis compared to that expected with conventional therapy.

| Generic Name | Brand Name |
|---|---|
| hydralazine | Apresoline |

Side effects of hydralazine can include headaches, rapid heartbeat, and joint pain.

## 47. What kind of medication is BiDil®?

BiDil® is an orally administered nitric oxide-enhancing medicine. BiDil® is a combination of two drugs, isosorbide dinitrate and hydralazine hydrochloride, that dilate arteries and veins. This combination therapy has been recently approved for treatment of CHF in African-American patients. In a trial of 1,050 African-American patients with CHF, BiDil® was effective in decreasing symptoms when it was added to standard therapy of diuretics, a beta blocker, and an ACE inhibitor (or angiotensin receptor blocker). The results of the study showed patients treated with BiDil® had improved survival and functional status, as well as prolonged the time to hospitalization.

## 48. What are beta blockers?

Beta blockers are a class of drugs that reduce the amount of work the heart does and decrease irregular heartbeats. Beta blockers work by "blocking" the effects of adrenaline on your body. As a result, they decrease the heart's need for blood and oxygen by reducing its workload. Their effect on nerve impulses also helps to prevent irregular heartbeats (arrhythmias). (See question 87 for more details.) Beta blockers are used in heart failure with normal ejection fraction as well as in low-output heart failure.

Some common brands of beta blockers are:

| Generic Name | Brand Name |
| --- | --- |
| sotalol | Betapace |
| timolol | Blocadren |
| nadolol | Corgard |
| propranolol | Inderal |
| bisoprolol | Zebeta |
| labetalol | Trandate |

Beta blockers may cause abnormally slow heart rate, breathing difficulty, or wheezing. They may hide symptoms of low blood sugar in diabetics, may exacerbate depression and asthma, and cause impotence.

## 49. I've heard there are new kinds of beta blockers available. Are they helpful in CHF?

One new medication recently approved by the Food and Drug Administration (FDA), carvedilol, was found to be of significant value to patients with mild to moderate CHF when used in conjunction with diuretics, ACE inhibitors, and digitalis. Clinical trials of this medication indicate that hospitalization time for CHF, as well as morbidity and mortality from the disease, was considerably reduced. Whether or not these results will apply to other beta blockers remains unclear and is an important issue, because newer agents such as carvedilol will be much more expensive than older ones such as metoprolol.

## 50. What is digitalis?

**Digitalis** is a medication derived from the foxglove plant and has been used to treat heart problems for over two centuries. The principal clinical uses currently are in the treatment of CHF and in the treatment of arrhythmias.

Digitalis works by increasing the pumping action of the heart by increasing the force of the heart's contractions. It also slows certain fast heart rhythms. As a result, the heart beats less frequently but more effectively, and more blood is pumped into the arteries. Digitalis is available in pill and liquid formulations as well as in a sterile injection form.

Digitalis has been a mainstay in the treatment of CHF due to its ability to increase the heart's contractility and decrease its workload. Digitalis is usually introduced after diuretics and ACE inhibitors. It has been shown to improve symptoms and morbidity, although not survival, in patients with a normal heart rhythm. Digitalis does appear to be of greatest benefit with more severe left ventricular dysfunction. Withdrawing digitalis in patients who are clinically stable on diuretics and ACE inhibitors has been shown to produce clinical deterioration. Therefore, patients should not stop taking digitalis without speaking with their doctor first.

Common brands of digitalis are:

| Generic Name | Brand Name |
|---|---|
| digitalis | Lanoxicaps |

**Digitalis**

Also known as **digoxin**. A medication that makes the heart pump more strongly and may also help control certain types of irregular heartbeats. Digitalis drugs are medicines made from a type of foxglove plant (*Digitalis purpurea*) that has a stimulating effect on the heart. Digitalis drugs are used to treat heart problems such as CHF and irregular heartbeat.

| digitalis | Lanoxin |
| digitalis | Lanoxin Elixir Pediatric |
| digitalis | Lanoxin Injection |
| digitalis | Lanoxin Injection Pediatric |

## 51. What are the side effects of digitalis?

In addition to its effects on the heart, digitalis may cause nausea, vomiting, loss of appetite, diarrhea, confusion, and new heartbeat irregularities. Digitalis toxicity can occur in any patient although the elderly and those with hypothyroidism are particularly prone.

## 52. What are blood thinners?

Although they are called blood thinners (anticoagulants), these medicines do not really thin your blood. Instead, they decrease the blood's ability to clot. Decreased clotting keeps fewer harmful blood clots from forming and from blocking blood vessels. Using blood thinners reduces your risk for heart attacks, strokes, and blood clots in the legs (called *phlebitis*, deep venous thrombosis, or DVTs).

Your doctor may prescribe a blood thinner if you have had a heart valve replaced or if you have atrial fibrillation, a history of DVTs, or CHF.

Blood thinners may be prescribed to treat a blood clot in the leg. They keep the blood clot from getting bigger, but do not break up the clots that have already formed. Blood thinners can be given as an injection under the skin into a vein or can be taken as a pill.

Blood thinners such as *heparin* are injected by a needle into your bloodstream. Heparin works quickly (within

*Blood thinners may be prescribed to treat a blood clot in the leg.*

minutes) to decrease clotting in the blood. The oral anticoagulants require several doses to take effect. Therefore, when the need for anticoagulation is emergent, doctors will give heparin but will treat with oral anticoagulants at the same time. The heparin maintains a level of anticoagulation immediately, while the oral anticoagulant reaches its therapeutic level after several days. When the oral anticoagulants have reached a therapeutic level, the intravenous heparin will be stopped. A new form of heparin (called low molecular weight heparin) may be prescribed for you to take at home under your doctor's supervision.

Common blood thinners are:

| Generic Name | Brand Name |
| --- | --- |
| warfarin | Coumadin |
| anisinidione | Miradon |
| (low molecular weight heparins) | |
| dalteparin | Fragmin |
| enoxaparin | Lovenox |

## 53. What are the side effects of blood thinners?

All blood thinners (anticoagulants) can result in unintended bleeding. Although this usually is manifested with only mild bruising, serious complications such as bleeding in the stomach, intestines, and the brain are possible. Blood thinners are lifesaving drugs and can be used safely, but they need frequent monitoring to make sure that you have neither unintended clotting nor unintended bleeding.

Less serious but more common complications of anticoagulants include:

• Bloating and gas

- Diarrhea
- Upset stomach or throwing up
- Feeling less hungry

## 54. What are some other drugs that are used to treat CHF?

Other drugs that are sometimes used to treat CHF include:

*Brain natriuretic peptide (BNP)* is a small peptide produced in the left ventricle and is released when the left ventricle experiences dilation or increased pressure. When BNP is released into the bloodstream, it causes the blood pressure to drop and reduces the strain on the heart, thus causing salts and water to be excreted by the kidneys. Scientists have been able to make BNP in the lab, and now patients can be treated with BNP as a method of treating CHF. The new medication is called nesiritide (brand name Natrecor). It is chemically identical to a naturally occurring peptide that the heart produces to try to relieve the symptoms of heart failure. Natrecor is used to rapidly reduce the elevated pressures within the heart and to improve shortness of breath. Use of Natrecor has been associated with side effects, such as low blood pressure, dizziness, and lightheadedness. If any of these symptoms occurs, please alert your health care provider immediately.

*Tumor Necrosis Factor–Alpha (TNF-α)* is a protein produced in the body and has an important role in the functioning of the immune system. TNF-α works to increase inflammation and fight infection. When released into the bloodstream, TNF-α can reduce the contractility of heart muscles and lead to dilation of the heart chambers (called *cardiac remodeling*). Heart

*Brain natriuretic peptide (BNP)*

A small protein that is stored mainly in cardiac ventricular myocardium and may be responsive to changes in ventricular filling pressures. It has been shown to decrease the work of the heart, lower blood pressure, and increase the excretion of salt from the body.

Treatment

enlargement, in this setting, is associated with poor outcomes. High levels of TNF-α are found after heart damage. Studies have demonstrated that the risk of death in heart failure patients increases with higher levels of TNF-α. Tumor necrosis factor may play an etiologic role in idiopathic-dilated cardiomyopathy. For these reasons, inhibition of TNF-α appears to be a valid target for the improvement of heart failure.

Pentoxifylline suppresses TNF-α production and reportedly produces beneficial effects. Pentoxifylline is sold under the brand name Trental. Infliximab is a medication that binds to TNF-α and blocks its function. It is highly effective in treating other diseases that are mediated by TNF-α, such as rheumatoid arthritis. However, in preliminary studies, it has not been shown to improve CHF outcomes. Infliximab is currently not recommended for the treatment of CHF and may result in worsening of CHF symptoms in some patients.

*Erythropoietin* is a drug that stimulates the production of red blood cells. When a person is *anemic* (that is, they have fewer red blood cells than they should), the heart has to work harder to get enough oxygen to the tissues. Anemia can contribute to or worsen symptoms of CHF. Patients with severe, poorly controlled CHF and mild anemia might benefit from erythropoietin and supplemental iron to raise their blood level.

*Thiamine* deficiency is caused by the chronic use of high-dose loop diuretics. Patients can achieve an improved ejection fraction by taking supplemental thiamine.

## SURGICAL TREATMENT

### 55. Are pacemakers used to treat heart failure?

Yes. Because of the changes in the heart that occur with heart failure, patients with heart failure may experience irregular heartbeats also known as arrhythmias. A pacemaker can help manage these irregular heart rhythms when medicines no longer work. Pacemakers and their more modern cousins called *implantable cardiac devices* are considered a routine and effective treatment for some heart failure patients.

Pacemakers used to control heart rhythm have been around for more than 40 years. A pacemaker is a small device, run by a battery, that helps the heart beat in a

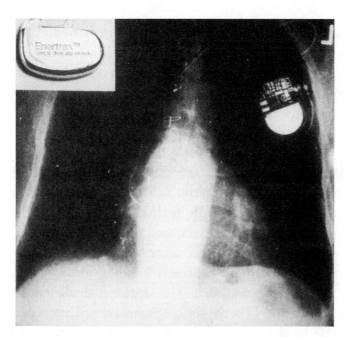

**Figure 2   X-ray with pacemaker present.**

*Pacemakers used to control heart rhythm have been around for more than 40 years.*

regular rhythm. Pacemakers can help pace the heart in cases of slow heart rate, fast and slow heart rate, or a (complete) blockage in the heart's electrical system.

A pacemaker can pace the heart's upper chambers (the atria), the lower chambers (the ventricles), or both. Pacemakers may also be used to stop the heart from triggering impulses or from sending extra impulses.

All pacemakers have two components. These are a pulse generator and leads. The pulse generator is a battery and a small computer that are connected to the heart via wires called leads. When the leads are connected, the computer monitors the heart's beat. When the heart slows down, the computer uses the battery to send a very small electrical pulse down the leads, which stimulates the heart to beat at a normal pace.

In the past, pacemakers had limited functions and were used only to speed up slowly beating hearts. The more sophisticated pacemakers of today can control the beating of each chamber of the heart or even shock the heart back to a normal rhythm when it has entered into a dangerous or even fatal type of arrhythmia.

With recent advances in computer miniaturization, longer lasting batteries, and an improved understanding of how the heart controls its rhythm, doctors and engineers have produced electronic marvels that both extend life and improve its quality. The size of the devices varies, depending on what each one does. Some are about the size of a wristwatch. The largest is smaller than a deck of cards. Like the simple pacemakers, doctors place these implantable devices under the skin of the upper chest. These implantable cardiac devices are now commonly used and have helped millions of patients.

**Cardiac resynchronization by biventricular pacemaker.** For some individuals, stimulating both the right and left ventricles improves the heart's ability to contract with more force, thereby improving symptoms and increasing the length of time they are able to exercise. A biventricular pacemaker affects both left and right chambers and may be beneficial for some of the approximately one quarter to one half of heart failure patients whose two ventricles do not beat in synchrony. You may be a candidate for this special pacemaker if your electrocardiogram and echocardiogram reveal specific characteristics, and you are still having symptoms of heart failure although you're receiving optimal medical therapy. In a 2002 study, one of these pacemakers was demonstrated to cut the risk of being rehospitalized for worsening heart failure in half. Some patients who used this type of device were taken off the transplant waiting list. This pacemaker also will help people with slow heart rates.

## 56. What are implantable cardioverter defibrillators (ICDs)?

Some patients with heart failure experience fast, irregular heartbeats. These heartbeats can just be annoying, make you weak and dizzy, or even result in death. Sometimes medicines are used to control these fast heart rates. When medicines do not work, doctors can implant an **implantable cardioverter defibrillator (ICD)**.

An ICD is used in patients at risk for:

- Ventricular **tachycardia,** when the lower chambers of the heart independently beat faster than 100 beats per minute

**Implantable cardioverter defibrillator (ICD)**

An electronic device that is placed under your skin and connected to your heart. It monitors your heart rhythm and gives a shock to the heart if the rhythm gets too slow or too fast. The shock is able to change the rhythm back to normal.

**Tachycardia**

A rapid heartbeat.

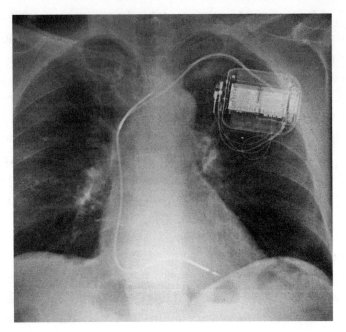

**Figure 3    X-ray of ICD.**

- Ventricular fibrillation, when the muscle fibers of the lower chambers of the heart contract in a fast, uncoordinated manner
- **Sudden cardiac death** caused by arrhythmias

**Sudden cardiac death**

An unexpected death due to heart disease; a death due to heart disease that occurs within 24 hours of the onset of symptoms.

The ICD is usually about the size of a pager. It constantly monitors the heart rhythm. When it detects a very fast, abnormal heart rhythm, it can give your heart a lifesaving shock to prevent cardiac arrest. Like the pacemakers, the ICD is composed of two parts: a battery that generates a pulse and a small computer that monitors the heart rate and determines when a electrical pulse is necessary to change the heart rhythm. The computer and battery are inserted under the skin near the collarbone and are connected to the heart with wires called leads. Newer ICD devices can also work like a pacemaker if your heart beats too slowly (bradycardias).

## 57. What are some mechanical devices that are used to improve pumping actions?

A growing array of heart devices and machines are changing the face of heart failure treatment. They have gained widespread acceptance for use as a bridge to transplant in patients who are on medications but still have severe symptoms and are awaiting a donor heart. Increasingly, though, doctors are exploring the possibility that such devices may be satisfactory treatments themselves, forestalling the need for a transplant altogether in some patients. These devices include the intra-aortic balloon pump, the left ventricular assist device, and the artificial heart.

## 58. What is an intra-aortic balloon pump?

The intra-aortic balloon pump (IABP) is helpful for maintaining heart function in people with left-side failure who are waiting for transplants as well as for those who develop a sudden and severe deterioration of heart function.

- The IABP is a thin balloon that is inserted into the artery in the leg and threaded up to the aorta.
- Its pumping action is generated by inflating and deflating the balloon within the aorta.

Usually, it is used only for short periods (20 to 72 hours), but some studies indicate that patients may be able to use it safely for somewhat longer periods (an average duration of 23 days in one study).

**Ventricular assist devices (VADs)**

These are machines that are implanted in the chest to help improve the pumping actions of the heart.

**Left ventricular assist device (LVAD)**

This is a mechanical device, connected to the heart, that aids the heart in pumping.

## 59. What is a ventricular assist device?

**Ventricular assist devices (VADs)** are machines that help improve pumping actions. A **left ventricular assist device (LVAD)** either takes over or assists the pumping role of the left ventricle, the heart's main pumping chamber. Newer LVADs are meant to be permanent in people with severe heart failure. It allows a person to be mobile, sometimes returning home to await a heart transplant.

Part of the device is implanted in your heart and abdomen and part remains outside your body. You carry the external part of the device on a belt around your waist or on a shoulder strap. Most LVADs right now have an electric pump, an electronic controller, an energy supply (usually a battery weighing about 8 pounds), and two tubes. One tube carries blood from your left ventricle into the device. The other tube takes blood pumped from the device into your aorta (artery) to be circulated throughout your body.

LVADs are used for patients whose heartbeat has slowed dangerously (bradycardia) to help take over the pumping action of the failing heart. Studies now suggest that in some people the use of an LVAD may allow some of the damaged heart muscle to heal, perhaps even helping some patients avoid heart transplants.

*LVADs are used for patients whose heartbeat has slowed dangerously.*

Until recently, these machines required that the patient remain in the hospital. Smaller battery-powered LVAD units, however, are allowing many patients to leave the hospital and are proving to be effective bridges to heart transplants in adults. For example, the HeartMate, a portable LVAD about the size of a portable CD player (2 in. by 4 in.), is implanted in the upper abdomen. The implanted device plugs into an external power base, which is employed when the patient is at rest to recharge the battery and provide continuous power.

The LVAD is known as the "bridge to transplantation" for patients who haven't responded to other treatments and are hospitalized with extreme systolic heart failure.

There are risks involved with many of these devices, including bleeding, blood clots, and right-side heart failure. Infections are a particular hazard.

## 60. What is an implantable artificial heart?

About 4,000 people in the United States await heart transplants each year. During a typical year, only about 2,500 donor hearts become available. Some of the 4,000 people awaiting heart transplants have nonreversible biventricular failure, a condition in which both the left and right sides of the heart are not functioning properly. These people could be candidates for an artificial heart.

Many types of artificial hearts are now being tested. In general, they are composed of two main parts. There is a smaller mechanical part that is connected to the person's heart or major arteries. It receives the blood and pumps it out of the mechanical heart into the aorta, the body's biggest artery. This internal part is connected to an air pump by hoses that exit the chest. Currently, the air pump is a washing machine–sized console that provides the power to the artificial heart. Manufacturers are working on smaller external pumps that can make the patient more mobile.

Although these devices help many patients successfully wait for a heart transplant, they are not without problems. In one study, 72 percent of those in the study developed infection. Other complications from artificial hearts include bleeding in the chest and lungs, strokes, and device malfunctions. Though researchers have been working on artificial hearts that could permanently replace diseased hearts, there are no such devices approved for permanent use.

The artificial heart is like a safety net for some patients, making them a better candidate for transplantation. The goal is to improve blood function, as well as lung and kidney function. They are intended as a temporary aid for patients with severe heart failure, unresponsive to maximal medical therapy, who are not expected to live longer than 30 days.

## 61. How are angioplasty and coronary bypass surgery used to treat CHF?

Patients with heart failure and severe coronary artery disease often benefit from angioplasty or bypass surgery. The surgery increases blood flow to the heart muscle. This may enhance the heart's pumping action and help to relieve symptoms.

Angioplasty is a catheter-based technique that does not require open-heart surgery. Specially trained cardiologists insert a small tube or catheter that has a balloon in its tip into an artery in the arm or groin. The catheter is threaded along the artery into the heart and then into the coronary artery. The cardiologist advances the balloon tip into an area of blockage or narrowing and the balloon is inflated. This opens the artery and allows blood to flow to the muscle.

The most common surgery for heart failure is bypass surgery. Your doctor will determine if your heart failure is caused by coronary artery disease and if you have blockages that can be "grafted" or bypassed. Although surgery is riskier for people with heart failure, new strategies before, during, and after surgery have reduced the risks and improved outcomes.

Even patients with coronary artery disease and very low ejection fraction can still benefit from bypass surgery, according to researchers from the VA Boston Healthcare System. The researchers say such patients now have options, especially patients who are considered too old or for other reasons do not qualify for a heart transplant. Despite the high risk of this patient population, studies show that the outcomes are good.

Victoria's comment:

*I was diagnosed with coronary artery disease and had three of my coronary arteries bypassed. This has improved my chest pain and seemed to improve my ejection fraction somewhat. I thought the surgery was going to hurt a lot, but it didn't. It took me a couple of months to get back into my regular routine, but I feel better than before the surgery. I am less short of breath when I do a lot of walking.*

## 62. How does heart–valve surgery improve CHF?

Diseases of the heart valves can be a common cause of heart failure. During valve surgery, the valves may be either repaired or replaced. In appropriate patients, valve surgery may significantly reduce the severity of heart failure and improve quality of life.

*Diseases of the heart valves can be a common cause of heart failure.*

**Mitral valve**

A heart valve. It lies between the left ventricle and the left atrium in the heart.

In a study of 92 patients with severe (Class III or Class IV) heart failure and faulty valves, reconstruction of the heart's **mitral valve** drastically improved heart function, and all patients were able to be reclassified as Class I or Class II patients. For more information read questions 83, 84, and 85.

## 63. What are ventricular remodeling procedures?

Ventricular remodeling procedures are complex heart surgeries. During the surgery, the chest is opened and the heart is stopped. The patient is placed on a "bypass pump" while the surgeon works. These procedures change the size and shape of the left ventricle in an attempt to improve the heart's performance.

## 64. What is a partial left ventriculectomy?

**Batista procedure**

Also called partial left ventriculectomy; a surgical procedure to remodel the left ventricle.

This procedure is also called the **Batista procedure**, after its inventor Dr. Randas Batista, a Brazilian heart surgeon, who developed this technique. When performing this procedure, a section of the left ventricular wall is removed. The remaining free edges are repositioned and sewed together. The mitral valve is also repaired or replaced. This type of ventricular remodeling may allow some patients with dilated cardiomyopathy to avoid a heart transplant.

The procedure is not beneficial for people whose heart failure developed from coronary artery disease or a heart attack and is not done very often. Complication rates are very high and only about one third of patients experience any benefit from it. The results of studies on long-term improvement from this procedure are mixed to date. Because of this, the Batista procedure has fallen out of favor with both cardiologists and heart surgeons.

## 65. What is a surgical anterior ventricular endocardial restoration?

This procedure is also called the SAVER or **Dor procedure** after its inventor, Dr. Vicent Dor of Monaco. When a heart attack occurs, a part of the heart muscle dies and a scar forms. The scarred area is thin and can bulge out with each beat. The bulging thin area is called an *aneurysm*. An aneurysm in the left ventricle decreases the ability of the heart to pump blood and heart failure occurs.

Like the Batista procedure discussed in question 64, the Dor procedure involves the removal of heart tissue to optimize the size and shape of the heart and to improve function. When heart failure occurs after a heart attack, the surgeon may choose to combine bypass surgery and/or valve repair with removal of the dead area of heart muscle or the aneurysm. After this surgery, most people's hearts pump better and they have fewer heart failure symptoms. An early study found that 85 percent of patients who had the surgery did not need to return to the hospital during an 18-month follow-up period.

## 66. What is a dynamic cardiomyoplasty?

Dynamic cardiomyoplasty is an experimental treatment that has been useful in carefully selected patients with congestive heart failure. Long-term and larger studies are still needed to prove that it is beneficial.

This procedure requires the surgeon to detach one end of a muscle from the patient's back and wrap it around

**Dor procedure**
A surgical procedure to make a dilated left ventricle smaller and more efficient.

Treatment

*The first heart transplants were performed in the late 1960s.*

the ventricles of the heart. After a few weeks, these re-located muscles are conditioned with a pacemaker to behave and beat as if they were heart muscles.

Initial tests indicate that the procedure benefits the failing heart in many ways, including improving systolic pressure, limiting dilation of the heart, reducing heart muscle stress, and possibly reversing unwanted cardiac remodeling.

In short-term studies, there have been problems with heart rhythm disturbances and in conditioning the re-located muscles. One study was stopped because of no determined difference in survival rates in patients with or without this procedure.

Additional experience indicated that it was the re-straining effect of the muscle wrap on the weakened heart that may have provided key benefits, so surgeons are now investigating cardiac support devices that cradle the heart in a mesh-like support as a possible new surgical avenue.

## 67. What is a heart transplantation?

The first heart transplants were performed in the late 1960s, but it was not until the use of anti-rejection medicines in the 1980s that the procedure became an accepted operation. Today, heart transplantation provides hope for a select group of patients who would otherwise die of heart failure.

Candidates for heart transplantation must meet several criteria before they are eligible for surgery. The patients should have severe heart failure symptoms, usually NYHA Class IV on maximal medical therapy. They should have no serious medical problems outside of their heart failure, and they must have a life expectancy of less than 1 year without a transplant.

Traditionally, heart transplants are performed only on more robust patients and patients under 60. About 76 percent of transplant patients are male and 85.4 percent are white. Studies published in 1998 and 2000 suggest that older and sicker patients may achieve the best benefits. In fact, a study of almost 900 patients found that transplantation increased survival only for the sickest of patients.

While the risks of this procedure are high, the 2-year survival rate is about 78 percent and after 5 years it ranges from 50 percent to over 70 percent. In general, the highest risk factors for death 3 or more years after a transplant operation are coronary artery disease and the adverse effects (infection and certain cancers) of immunosuppressive drugs used in the procedure. The rejection rates in older people appear to be similar to those of younger patients.

A significant problem with heart transplants is that there simply are not enough hearts available. In the United States each year, only about 2,500 heart transplants are performed, while 25,000–50,000 people die each year while waiting for a heart transplant. Some people with heart failure do become candidates for transplantation, but most never do. Not all transplant units accept Medicare patients.

## 68. What is myocardial replacement therapy?

Myocardial replacement therapy is a biologic treatment rather than a pharmacologic treatment for heart failure. This investigational therapy uses stem cells to grow new heart cells in a damaged heart. The stem cells are taken from the patient's own bone marrow and are implanted into the heart either by direct injection into the heart muscle with a needle or catheter or by infusing the cells into the heart itself.

Experiments on animals and humans show that not only do these stem cells grow into heart muscle cells; they also contract normally along with the other "native" heart muscle cells. A concern is that these new cells appear to cause irregular heartbeats (arrhythmias) in experimental subjects that require treatment with medication or an implantable cardioverter defibrillator.

Although this therapy appears to be a feasible approach to heart repair, there are many technical issues that scientists must address before it becomes a viable treatment. These technical issues include how to grow the stem cells in sufficient numbers to affect meaningful replacement of heart tissue, when to use this therapy after a heart attack or other heart muscle damage, and what is the best method for delivering these cells into the heart muscle.

## 69. Is alternative or complementary medicine helpful in CHF?

Alternative medicine and complementary medicine are terms that are often used interchangeably and will be used as such in this discussion.

*Alternative medicine* is a mixed group of practices that include the areas of hygiene, diagnosis, and treatment of many diseases. The theoretical bases of alternative medicine diverge from those of modern scientific medicine and are not generally accepted by modern physicians. Alternative medicine has failed to gain acceptance because these practices currently lack a plausible scientific basis as well as any medical studies demonstrating their safety and efficacy.

Alternative medicine may come from some of the following sources:

- Religious
- Cultural
- Supernatural, magical, or cultist
- Naive, illogical, or false understandings of anatomy, physiology, pathology, or pharmacology
- Fraud and exploitation of the sick and hopeless

Any treatment that is outside the traditional medicine or practice of your primary health system can be considered alternative medicine. A treatment that is alternative in one culture may be traditional in another. For example, acupuncture is a well-accepted system of treatment that has been practiced in China for more than 5000 years, yet in the United States, it is considered an alternative medicine.

Practitioners of Western (allopathic) medicine are closely monitored and regulated in the United States, having to undergo rigorous training and testing as well as licensing by state and federal authorities. The facilities of modern practitioners, such as hospitals, surgical centers, and dialysis units undergo similar scrutiny and licensing. Complementary medicine practitioners and their therapies are rarely, if ever, subject to this level of testing and regulation in the United States. Therefore, patients who seek these therapies cannot be confident in the abilities of the practitioners to safely practice their remedies.

Although complementary medicine offers the ability for people to take greater responsibility for their own health care, it also subjects its supporters to the risks of taking charge of their own health care. While mainstream medicine is not perfect in many ways, it does remain an enormous resource of knowledge and expertise. It is highly unlikely that consumers or practitioners who have lesser training will be as effective over the long run.

The greatest risk involved associated with using complementary medicine is that it may be used instead of a necessary or possibly lifesaving treatment from a practitioner of conventional medicine. It is always best to get as much information as possible about new therapies, be they complementary or conventional treatments. Then make an informed decision in consultation with your primary health professional.

Like traditional medicines, alternative, complementary, or herbal medicines are not free of side effects. Other risks associated with complementary therapies include the potential for dangerous interactions with conventional therapies, a lack of evidence on the effectiveness of many complementary therapies, and the fact that the expense of many complementary therapies may not be covered by health insurance.

The growing consumer interest in alternative medicine has expanded the market for a wide range of products from acupuncture to the multiple dietary supplements which are now on the market. Supplements are popular, but are they safe?

Since 1994 when Congress decided that dietary supplements should be regulated as if they were foods, they are now assumed to be safe unless the Food and Drug Administration can demonstrate that they pose a significant risk to the consumer. Manufacturers are not legally required to provide specific information about safety before marketing their products. Further, some supplements may interfere with your other CHF medications. Therefore, supplements should be used with caution and only after discussions with your treating physician.

## 70. What are some alternative medicine treatments for CHF?

The following are some alternative medicine treatments along with their health claims. The alternative treatments listed below have been recommended by alternative medicine practitioners for the treatment of CHF. The benefits of these therapies are not supported by scientific studies. Alternative treatments are generally not recommended by cardiologists. You should discuss these therapies with your physician before trying any.

- **Antioxidants**: The following is a list of antioxidants that are reported to decrease "oxidative damage" to the heart.
  - Vitamin C
  - Vitamin E
  - Selenium
  - Coenzyme Q10 (increases oxygenation of tissue, including heart muscle)
- **Homocysteine metabolism**:
  - Folic acid
  - Vitamin B6
  - Vitamin B12
  - Betaine
- **Magnesium**: A mild vasodilator (dilates blood vessels)

- **Taurine**: Helps your heart work more efficiently
- **Carnitine**: Important in fatty acid metabolism, increases efficiency of cardiac function

**Essential fatty acids** are advertised to work as anti-inflammatory agents. Fatty acids are the building materials of fats. Most fatty acids can be produced in your body; however, the essential fatty acids need to be part of your diet, because they cannot be produced by your body. There are two essential fatty acids, called alpha linolenic acid and linoleic acid. Alpha linolenic acid, also known as the omega 3 fatty acid, is found in flax seed, walnuts, and canola oil. Linoleic acid, also known as omega 6 fatty acid, is found in soy, sunflower seeds, corn oil, and most nuts.

**Diet:**
- Garlic, ginger, and onions all have a beneficial effect on circulation.
- Increase fiber (especially water soluble), fruits, vegetables
- Vegetarian sources of protein
- Increase potassium and decrease sodium in the diet

**Herbs:** Herbs may be used as dried extracts (capsules, powders, teas), glycerites (glycerine extracts), or tinctures (alcohol extracts). The following is a list of herbs with their benefit claims. These have been recommended by alternative medicine practitioners for CHF. These claims have not been supported by scientific evidence.

- Hawthorne *(Crataegus monogyna)*: Increases blood vessel integrity
- Mistletoe *(Viscum album)*: Protects against high blood pressure and hardening of the arteries, historically for exhaustion and nervousness

- Linden (*Tilia cordata*): Historically used to lower blood pressure
- Rosemary *(Rosmarinus officinalis)*: Increases coronary artery blood flow, used to stimulate digestion and relieve nervous tension
- Motherwort *(Leonurus cardiaca)*: Regulates heart rhythm
- Dandelion *(Taraxacum officinale)*: Potassium-sparing diuretic
- Indian tobacco *(Lobelia inflata)*: Helps reduce spasm, stimulates respiratory function, used in smoking cessation. May be toxic if used above recommended doses.
- Lily of the valley *(Convallaria majalis)*: Specific for cardiac insufficiency; exceeding recommended doses may lead to nausea, vomiting, headache, stupor. Use no more than 30 drops per day.
- Horsetail herb *(Equisetum arvense)*: Diuretic

**Acupuncture:** May be helpful for increasing circulation and cardiac strength. Acupuncture may also help patients quit smoking. Acupuncture has been shown to decrease breathlessness, increase walking distance, and improve lung function in chronic obstructive pulmonary disease (COPD).

**Massage**: May help increase lymphatic drainage and reduce swelling.

**Biofeedback**: Biofeedback is a training model that uses instruments and computers as tools to aid in relaxation and improve health and reach optimal performance. Biofeedback instruments use electronic sensors to pick up signals from the body and to feed the results of the measurement back to the individual so that they can learn to consciously control their body's functions.

*Acupuncture may also help patients quit smoking.*

Combined with stress management skills, the biofeedback component allows both the facilitator and the client to experiment with various stress management techniques and to fine-tune them optimally for the individual. Biofeedback converts vague feelings into hard, observable information. Learning occurs much more rapidly than without the benefits of the instant feedback loop. Biofeedback has been used to reduce stress and relieve anxiety in many studies. Research in its use in CHF is lacking.

**Yoga**: Most people who try yoga find that it increases flexibility and reduces stress. Studies demonstrating beneficial effects of yoga on CHF patients are lacking. Keep in mind that any exercise plan should be discussed with your physician before starting.

**REMINDER**: Before you try any of these therapies, discuss their possible benefits and side effects with your health professional. Let your doctor know if you are already using any such therapies.

# PART FIVE

# Rehabilitation

What is cardiac rehabilitation?

Is cardiac rehabilitation helpful
for patients with CHF?

*More...*

## 71. What is cardiac rehabilitation?

Cardiac rehabilitation is a structured program of exercise and education run by a team of experts in heart disease and aimed at improving the patient's quality of life while extending the length of life. This is accomplished through electrocardiographic monitoring, clinical observation, and assessment of signs and symptoms. Supervised cardiac rehabilitation results in early-problem detection, leading to improvements in medical care. Early detection and resolution of medical problems help to prevent cardiac complications that would require extended outpatient and inpatient treatments.

## 72. What are the goals of a cardiac rehabilitation program?

The goals of a cardiac rehabilitation program should include:

- Detecting signs and symptoms of heart disease at rest
- Assuring safety during physical activity by monitoring ECG, heart rate, blood pressure, and symptomatic responses to exercise
- Improving adherence to the exercise, diet, smoking cessation, and stress reduction prescriptions
- Increasing exercise tolerance
- Decreasing symptoms of disease
- Decreasing mortality
- Reducing negative emotional effects of disease
- Enhancing self-confidence to achieve or resume an active lifestyle

## 73. What are the components of a cardiac rehabilitation program?

All cardiac rehabilitation programs should be supervised by a cardiac physician, managed by heart care professionals, and offer a standard group of services. A good cardiac rehabilitation program focuses on the needs of the individual; therefore, although the overall program may have a wide variety of standard programs, each patient's program will have different emphases and different components.

*A good cardiac rehabilitation program focuses on the needs of the individual.*

**Rehabilitation**

Behavioral factors, such as poor compliance with nutritional and pharmacological treatment regimens, frequently contribute to exacerbations of CHF in the elderly. In part, noncompliance may be due to the difficult-to-follow medication schedules prescribed by health care providers. It is estimated that 20 to 58 percent of patients with CHF are noncompliant with medications.

Noncompliance is a major cause of unnecessary hospitalization. Of patients hospitalized with heart failure, 27 percent were rehospitalized within 90 days due to dietary and/or medication noncompliance. Readmission rates for patients 65 years and older with CHF approach 50 percent. Factors that may contribute include social isolation, poor compliance with medications, and poor diet. Programs providing case management for CHF have been effective. An effective rehabilitation program will address these issues.

According to the American Heart Association, the principles of cardiac rehabilitation include:

- A thorough medical evaluation, with an emphasis on maximizing the benefits of existing medications
- A supervised program of aerobic and resistance training exercises
- Education and programs on how to change the patient's lifestyle to better manage acquired risk factors, such as:
  - High blood pressure
  - Smoking
  - High blood cholesterol
  - Physical inactivity
  - A diet high in salt, calories, and fat
- Stress management programs
- Counseling for depression
- Nutritional counseling
- Lending emotional support
- Providing vocational guidance to enable the patient to return to work
- Supplying information on physical limitations

## 74. What does a cardiac rehabilitation program accomplish?

Cardiac rehabilitation produces physiological, metabolic, and psychological benefits. The most important beneficial health outcomes are a reduction in mortality, improvement in the number of cardiac events, improvement in symptoms, increased exercise tolerance, improvement in blood lipids, increased smoking cessation, and improved psychosocial outcomes.

Cardiac rehabilitation also reduces hospitalizations and increases productivity of those who successfully complete them. This saves the patient and the health care system money.

## 75. How long does the rehabilitation last?

The number of rehabilitation sessions needed for a specific patient to achieve his or her rehabilitation goals remains a matter of clinical judgment by the physician and cardiac rehabilitation team. The length of cardiac rehabilitation will vary with the patient's condition and ability to comply with the rigors of the program. Some factors that may affect the duration of the rehab program include:

- Stability of the patient
- Acuity of the disease
- Patient's ability to adhere to medical and behavioral advice

For most patients who are likely to benefit from cardiac rehabilitation, 8 to 12 weeks of cardiac rehabilitation is sufficient to meet the goals outlined. Patients who fail to demonstrate progress and continue to have adverse signs and symptoms may require additional sessions. As patients progress, they can move to an at-home or group phase with less monitoring. By the end of the program, patients should be ready to maintain a healthier lifestyle on their own.

## 76. Is cardiac rehabilitation helpful for patients with CHF?

Yes, cardiac rehabilitation has been well studied and found useful in patients with many types of heart diseases, including congestive heart failure, coronary artery disease, and after heart attacks and bypass and valve surgery as well as heart transplantation. A strong body of scientific evidence exists that establishes the benefits of cardiac rehabilitation. A consensus is growing among health professionals that cardiac rehabilitation should be considered a standard of care, not only because of its defined medical benefit, but also because it is cost effective, reduces disability, improves productivity, and reduces health care costs.

Victoria's comment:

*I participated in one of these programs after I was diagnosed with CHF. I found it difficult to keep up with. I was short of breath and I've got arthritis in both knees that makes it difficult to exercise. I did feel better when I had just finished the program. I could walk further than before with less shortness of breath. Eventually, my knees started to hurt and I got lazy. I think the biggest help the rehab program gave me was, it let me know that exercise wasn't going to kill me. Now I know that I can walk around and get short of breath, but if I don't overdo it, I'll feel better after a short rest.*

## 77. What do I ask my doctor about cardiac rehabilitation?

Despite the known benefits of cardiac rehabilitation (rehab), only 15 percent of qualified patients participate in a program. Reasons for this include a lack of physician referral (especially among women and the elderly), poor patient motivation, logistical or lack of health insurance benefits and other financial constraints, or a combination of these factors.

Although you may have CHF and therefore should benefit from a rehab program, there may be good reasons that your doctor may not recommend cardiac rehab, such as other medical conditions that make exercise more dangerous than normal or that there are no rehabilitation programs in your area.

If a full-scale cardiac rehabilitation program is unavailable in your area or not right for you, there are alternatives. For example, although not everyone can participate in a monitored exercise program, almost everyone with heart disease or risk factors for heart disease would benefit from some form of risk factor assessment, activity counseling, and health education.

Home exercise training programs are beneficial in certain low-risk patient groups. They offer the advantages of convenience and low cost but lack the valuable elements of professional supervision, education, and group interaction.

Discuss with your doctor your interest in cardiac rehabilitation. He or she should be able to tell you about the availability of rehabilitation programs in your area and make a referral for you.

## 78. What happens after I finish the rehabilitation program?

It is expected that what you learn and practice during the program, you will continue in your daily life after the program ends. If you stop exercising after the program or stop taking your medications as directed, the improvements you have made will soon be lost. The rehabilitation staff will work with you to design a long-term plan of exercise. The staff will guide you in how and when to exercise at home. Many programs offer a "maintenance" plan so that you can continue to exercise with others and be supervised by professionals.

# PART SIX

# Heart Valves

What are the heart valves?

How can problems with the heart valves cause heart failure?

What causes valve disease?

*More . . .*

## 79. What are the heart valves?

While the myocardium or heart muscle is the workhorse of the heart, it is the heart valves that direct the flow of blood. Without properly functioning heart valves, the heart would fail in a matter of hours. Blood circulates through the human heart in only one direction. The heart valves open and close with each beat of the heart. When the heart pushes blood out of the atria or ventricles, the valves open to allow the outflow of blood. When the valves close, the blood cannot flow backward. The valves are round and have thin pliable flaps, called *leaflets*. The leaflets open and close in response to the changing pressure of the blood on either side of them.

The human heart has four valves. There is one valve to control the flow of blood for each chamber. Each heart valve is slightly different in size and character from the others and each has a different name.

The names of the heart valves are:

- **Mitral valve**
- **Aortic valve**
- **Tricuspid valve**
- **Pulmonic valve**

The heart's upper chambers are called *atria* and the lower chambers are called *ventricles*. Blood without oxygen returns from the body and flows into the right atrium. From there, it is forced through the tricuspid valve into the right ventricle beneath it. The right ventricle pumps the blood through the pulmonic valve and into the lungs while simultaneously closing the tricuspid valve. Therefore, the pulmonic valve opens to allow the blood to flow into the lung and the tricuspid valve closes to stop blood from flowing back into the right atrium.

**Mitral valve**

A valve in the heart that lies between the left atrium (LA) and the left ventricle (LV). The mitral valve and the tricuspid valve are known as the atrioventricular valves, because they lie between the atria and the ventricles of the heart.

**Aortic valve**

The heart valve between the left ventricle and the aorta.

**Tricuspid valve**

A valve in the heart that controls the flow of blood between the right atrium and the right ventricle.

**Pulmonic valve**

A valve with three cusps. It lies between the right ventricle and the pulmonary artery.

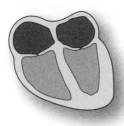

**Figure 4-a**  This figure shows the heart in late systole. The atria are full but the ventricles are empty.

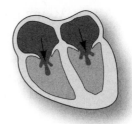

**Figure 4-b**  In early diastole, the mitral and tricuspid valves open, allowing a large amount of blood to rush into the ventricles. This is the rapid filling phase of diastole.

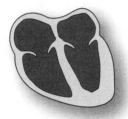

**Figure 4-c**  In mid-diastole, the ventricles are full. Notice that the ventricular walls, however, are not distended in any way.

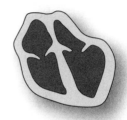

**Figure 4-d**  The atrial contraction allows an extra amount of blood to enter the ventricles, causing them to stretch and overfill. The slight stretch in the ventricular muscle caused by the atrial kick will maximize stroke volume and cardiac output.

**Diagram of heart during systole and diastole.**

Although the valves have different names on the left side of the heart, they operate in the same way as the right-sided valves. Oxygen-rich blood returning from the lungs flows into the left atrium. When the atrium contracts, this blood is forced through the mitral valve into the left ventricle beneath it. When the left ventricle contracts, the mitral valve closes, stopping the backflow of blood. At the same time, the aortic valve opens, allowing blood to flow into the rest of the body. When the left ventricle has finished its contraction, the aortic valve closes, stopping the backflow of blood, and the mitral valve opens, allowing blood from the left atrium to fill the left ventricle.

At any given time in the cardiac cycle, two valves are open, allowing blood to flow, and two valves are closed, stopping the backflow of blood. When your doctor listens to your heart, he or she can usually hear the opening and closing of the valves.

## 80. How can problems with the heart valves cause heart failure?

Two types of problems can disrupt blood flow through the valves: regurgitation or stenosis. Either type of problem can cause your heart to work harder, and eventually fail.

## 81. What is heart-valve regurgitation?

Valve regurgitation is also known as valve insufficiency or **valve incompetence**. These terms simply mean that the valve is leaking. Blood is not leaking outside the heart or arteries, but is allowed to flow backward into the heart. Regurgitation happens either when a valve does not close properly or the valve develops a hole or tear in it. In both these situations, the valve cannot form an effective seal against the flow of blood, thus allowing the blood to leak backward. When any blood is allowed to flow backward, less blood is able to flow forward. The greater the regurgitation, the harder the heart has to work to get the same amount of blood to the body. Initially, small amounts of backward flow or regurgitation may not be noticed by the patient. The heart responds to this increased stress by getting larger and more muscular, making it able to push more blood forward. Over time, the heart becomes stretched out or dilated. It looks and acts more like a bag than a pump. Eventually, the dilated heart is unable to meet the demands of the body. The patient then begins to feel the symptoms of heart failure.

*Valve incompetence*

When one of the heart valves no longer functions normally; either decreasing the flow of blood in one direction, called stenosis, or allowing blood to flow backward, called incompetence.

## 82. What is heart-valve stenosis?

**Heart-valve stenosis** occurs when the valve leaflets do not open wide enough and only a small amount of blood can flow through the valve. People can be born with a narrow valve opening or the valve leaflets can become thickened, stiffened, or even fuse together due to infection or disease. A smaller opening in the valve means that if the heart is going to keep circulating the same amount of blood, then it will have to either beat faster or beat harder to push more blood out. When the valve leaflets become very thick and stiff, the valve not only doesn't open well, it doesn't close well either; that is, the valve develops not only stenosis, but regurgitation as well. The increased workload on the heart results in heart failure if the valve problem is not corrected.

**Heart-valve stenosis**

A narrowing of the opening of a heart valve. This restricts the outflow of blood and can lead to heart failure.

**Heart Valves**

## 83. What causes valve disease?

Before doctors started giving their patients antibiotics, rheumatic fever was the single biggest cause of valve disease. Today, the cause of valve disease is most likely linked to one of the following:

- **Infective endocarditis**: An infection in the lining of the heart's walls (called the endocardium) and its valves.
- **Coronary artery disease**: The heart valves are anchored to the heart muscle. Abnormalities of the heart muscle because of poor blood flow from an obstructed coronary artery can affect how the valves function.
- **Myxomatous degeneration**: Myxomatous degeneration is a cardiac condition that is characterized by replacement of the tough connective tissue in the heart valve with softer gelatinous material. This weakens the valve and makes it floppy. The floppy valve does

*Many people with valve disease have no symptoms initially.*

not effectively control the flow of blood through the heart. Myxomatous degeneration occurs most often in the elderly and commonly affects the mitral valve.

- **Calcific degeneration**: A buildup of calcium on the aortic or mitral valves, which causes the valves to thicken.
- **Congenital defect of the valves**: Irregularly shaped, narrowed, or even absent valves can occur at birth. These abnormal valves may result in heart failure, even in an infant. Alternatively, they may function well until the patient enters adulthood. More exercise and a larger body put more of a strain on the heart and heart failure develops when the patient is in his 40's or 50's.

## 84. How is valve disease diagnosed?

Many people with valve disease have no symptoms initially. The problem may first be noticed by a physician during a routine physical exam. Using a stethoscope, the doctor can listen to the heart and hear the valves opening and closing. Abnormal clicking, or murmurs, can signal valve disease and should prompt further evaluation with some of the tests listed here.

- An electrocardiogram (EKG or ECG) can be used to find out if your ventricles or atria are enlarged. An EKG can also determine if you have an irregular heartbeat (arrhythmia).
- A chest X-ray can show if your heart is enlarged. This can happen if a valve is not working properly.
- An echocardiogram is a test that examines your heart using sound waves. These sound waves can produce a picture of the thickness of your heart's walls, your valves' shape and action, as well as the size of the valve openings. An advanced version,

called *Doppler echocardiography* or more simply called *ultrasound*, can be used to find out how severe the abnormality of the valves is.

- Coronary angiography is a part of cardiac catheterization, a test that involves the doctor putting a catheter into your heart and injecting dye into it. Using X-rays to see the dye, it lets doctors see your heart as it is pumping. The doctors can see how blood flows in and out of the heart and how well the valves are working. Angiography can help identify a narrowed valve or any backflow of blood. This test also helps doctors decide if you need surgery.
- Magnetic resonance imaging (MRI) technology uses magnetic fields to examine the heart and its surrounding structures. New machines can get images quickly and can give a three-dimensional picture of your heart and valves.

## 85. How is valve disease treated?

Ultimately, failed or failing heart valves are repaired or replaced. Since heart-valve surgery can be a risky procedure, people who do not have any symptoms or only minimal symptoms are not candidates for surgery. People with mild to moderate symptoms of heart-valve disease can be prescribed medications that treat the symptoms. If the underlying valve condition gets worse or if the symptoms become hard to control with medicine, then a surgical procedure is indicated.

**Medication for heart-valve disease** Medicines are given to treat the most common problems of valvular heart disease, symptoms of fatigue, shortness of breath, and irregular heartbeats. Medications can improve symptoms, but do not cure the diseased valves. The following medicines are commonly prescribed.

- **Digitalis** helps your heart to pump and eases some of the symptoms of valve disease.
- **Diuretics** or "water pills" can lower the salt and fluid levels in your body. Diuretics also reduce swelling and ease the workload on your heart.
- **Anticoagulant medicines** such as heparin and coumadin prevent blood clots, especially in patients who have had heart-valve surgery and have a prosthetic valve made of synthetic material.
- **Beta blockers** control your heart rate and lower your blood pressure.
- **ACE inhibitors** lower your blood pressure and help to keep your heart from overworking itself.

For a more in-depth discussion of these and other medications, see questions 39–54.

**Catheter surgery for heart-valve disease** In the past, all valve surgery required an open-heart procedure. Today, specialized cardiologists and surgeons can insert thin tubes (*catheters*) with a balloon tip into an artery in your arm or leg to fix some problems with heart valves. The catheter is advanced from the arm or leg into the heart. The balloon tip is placed between the leaflets of the valves. When the balloon is inflated, it pushes back any deposits along the edge of the valve, making the central area of the valve larger. The catheter and de-flated balloon are then removed from the valve. Often, the patient can be discharged the next day with im-proved symptoms. This procedure, called a *balloon valvuloplasty,* can be used to open narrowed tricuspid and pulmonary valves, a narrowed mitral valve, and on rare occasions, the aortic valve.

**Open-heart surgery for heart-valve disease** When medications can no longer control a patient's symptoms and a catheter procedure is either not indicated or has failed, doctors will suggest open-heart surgery. During surgery, valves may either be repaired or replaced. Because this surgery requires the doctors to open up the heart to fix the valve, the heart is stopped for a short time and a heart-lung machine must be used to circulate the blood. This machine pumps blood for the heart when the surgeons have stopped the heart to repair it. Repair may involve opening a narrowed valve by removing calcium deposits or reinforcing a valve that doesn't close properly. Surgeons replace valves that cannot be repaired. The diseased valve is removed and a replacement valve is put in its place.

Replacement valves are commonly either mechanical or biological. Mechanical valves are made from materials such as plastic, carbon, or steel. Biological valves are made from human or animal tissues.

Mechanical valves increase the risk of blood clots forming on the new valve. Patients with mechanical heart valves will need to take blood-thinning medicines for the rest of their lives. Biological valves often do not require blood-thinning medications. Newer hybrid valve types combine the best features of mechanical and biological valves and are now being used more commonly.

## 86. Why do I have to tell my dentist and other doctors that I have a problem with my heart valve?

If you have valve disease, even if you have no symptoms, you should always tell your dentist. Patients with diseased, poorly functioning, or replacement valves are at a high risk for developing infections after dental procedures and other surgical procedures, including

*Whenever you are giving a doctor or dentist your medical history, remember to tell him or her that you have valve disease.*

abdominal surgery, gynecological surgery, and urinary tract surgery. Colonoscopy also increases your risk of developing a valve infection. To prevent these infections, patients are given antibiotics before and after the procedures.

Whenever you are giving a doctor or dentist your medical history, remember to tell them if you have valve disease. If you have valve disease and do not take antibiotic medicine before a dental or surgical procedure, you may increase your risk of developing an infection in the inner lining of your heart. Endocarditis can rapidly deteriorate the valve and make it fail. Endocarditis is treated with high-dose intravenous antibiotics. If endocarditis is allowed to progress, a valve replacement may be necessary.

# PART SEVEN

# *Managing Your CHF*

What is an arrhythmia?

I thought low blood pressure was a good thing.
Why is my doctor concerned about my
low blood pressure?

Is depression common with CHF?

*More . . .*

*Palpitations are a common symptom that just about everyone experiences at one time or another.*

## 87. My cardiologist says that I have an arrhythmia. What is that?

An *arrhythmia* is an irregular heartbeat or any disorder of heart rate or rhythm. Arrhythmias are also called *irregular heartbeats, abnormal heart rhythms,* or *dysrhythmias.* They come in several varieties called *tachycardias* (the heartbeat is too fast), *bradycardias* (the heartbeat is too slow), and *"true" arrhythmias* (a disturbed rhythm).

These can often be felt as heart palpitations. Palpitations are a common symptom that just about everyone experiences at one time or another. Whether or not palpitations are of medical concern is ultimately determined by medical history, physical exam findings, and medical testing. Most people know when it is time to go to see the physician because the palpitations have become sustained and very uncomfortable or they are associated with another symptom such as shortness of breath, weakness, or fainting. CHF patients often have irregular heartbeats, much more than people the same age without CHF.

Any disruption of the normal electrical conduction system of the heart can cause an arrhythmia. Normally, the four chambers of the heart contract in a very specific, coordinated manner.

The signal for the heart to contract in a synchronized manner is an electrical impulse that begins in the *sinoatrial node* (also called the SA node), which is the body's natural pacemaker. The signal leaves the sinoatrial node and travels through the two atria, stimulating them to contract. Then the signal passes through an-

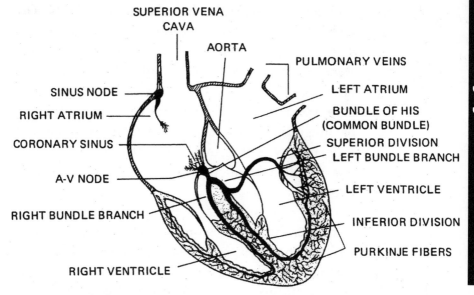

**Figure 5  Heart's electric conduction system.**

other node (the atrioventricular node or AV node) and finally travels through the ventricles and stimulates them to contract in synchrony.

Problems can occur anywhere along the conduction system, causing various arrhythmias. There can be a problem in the heart muscle itself, causing it to respond differently to the signal or causing the ventricles to contract independently of the normal conduction system. People at higher risk for arrhythmias and complications from arrhythmias include the following:

- Those who have a history of cardiac conditions such as coronary artery disease or heart-valve disorders
- Those with imbalances of blood chemistries
- Those who take medicines that stimulate or depress the heart conduction system, such as beta blockers, psychotropics, sympathomimetics, caffeine, amphetamines, and cocaine

*Arrhythmias cause the heart to beat less effectively.*

**Frequency of irregular heartbeats in patients with CHF** When doctors measure the heartbeats of CHF patients over several days (a test called a *Holter monitor*), they notice a high incidence of irregular heartbeats. Not only do a large number of patients have them, but these patients have many episodes of irregular heartbeats in a day. In one study, a dangerous type of arrhythmia, ventricular tachycardia, was recorded in 40 percent or more of the patient population.

Cardiac arrhythmias can make you feel sick, fatigued, give you chest pain, and if severe, they can cause death. Arrhythmias cause the heart to beat less effectively. A less-effective heart results in a decreased flow of blood to vital organs. Patients experience this lack of blood flow in symptoms such as increased anxiety, feelings of weakness, dizziness, and fainting. When the heart's pumping function is severely decreased for more than a few seconds, blood circulation is essentially stopped and organ damage (such as brain damage) may occur within a few minutes. A prolonged amount of arrhythmias can be life threatening.

Although any irregular heartbeat has the potential for causing problems, cardiologists list a few as being seriously life threatening. These arrhythmias include the following:

- Ventricular fibrillation
- Ventricular tachycardia that is rapid and sustained or results in an absent pulse
- Sustained episodes of other arrhythmias

Although not usually life threatening, other arrhythmias you may have heard the doctor mention are:

- Atrial fibrillation/flutter
- Multifocal atrial tachycardia
- Paroxysmal supraventricular tachycardia
- Wolff-Parkinson-White syndrome
- Sinus tachycardia
- Sinus bradycardia
- Bradycardia associated with heart block
- Sick sinus syndrome
- Ectopic heartbeat

**Treatment of arrhythmias in CHF patients** The treatment of cardiac arrhythmias is like the treatment of many diseases in medicine; that is, doctors attempt to "fix" the underlying problem, if possible; if not, they try to fix the symptoms.

When an underlying cause can be found, it usually stems from diseases of the coronary arteries or the heart muscle itself. Therefore, improving the blood supply to the heart, decreasing the heart's stress, and eliminating irritants to the heart (such as stimulant drugs or hormones like adrenaline) are all first priorities.

After this, doctors attempt to suppress fast heart rates by giving medications, such as beta blockers that slow down the heart. If the heart is beating too slowly, the rate can be increased by using pacemakers to provide the regular electrical stimulus that is missing in the diseased conduction system.

Implantable electrical devices, such as biventricular pacemakers, overdrive pacemakers, and implantable cardioverter defibrillators, can be used to coordinate all the heart chambers, regulate a fast heart rhythm, or even shock the heart if it stops beating. These devices are discussed in more detail in question 56.

## 88. I thought low blood pressure was a good thing. Why is my doctor concerned about my low blood pressure?

Low blood pressure is not a good thing, because it leads to poor blood circulation, dizziness, and fainting. Normal blood pressure is good. The misunderstanding about low blood pressure comes about because the doctor is often not clear in what he means when he discusses blood pressure with you. When the doctor takes your blood pressure with the arm cuff and meter (called a *sphygmomanometer*) and the blood pressure is high, what they would like is for your blood pressure to be lower but not "low." Most normal blood pressures fall in the range of 90/60 mm Hg to 130/80 mm Hg, but a significant change, even as little as 20 mm Hg, can cause problems for some people.

Blood pressure can be defined as the force of the blood against the walls of the blood vessels. Low blood pressure, also called *hypotension* by doctors, is an abnormal and serious condition. It is characterized by an amount of blood pressure that is insufficient to properly perfuse the heart, brain, and other vital organs. Low blood pressure is not a specific reading or number. For example, a blood pressure level that is borderline low for one person may be normal for another. The most important factor is how much the blood pressure changes.

**Causes of low blood pressure** In CHF patients, low blood pressure can be caused by many things. A sudden decrease in the heart's ability to pump can cause low blood pressure. A heart attack, an irregular heartbeat, or a decreased amount of oxygen in the blood can all impair the heart's ability to pump. A malfunction of a heart valve is another example of a problem that can lower the blood pressure. Low blood pressure can also occur because of the effects of medication. Diuretics decrease the amount of salt and water in your body. If you take too much diuretic, there may not be enough fluid in your body for the heart to pump and your blood pressure can drop. Similarly, too much of any blood pressure–lowering medication can decrease your blood pressure into the "low" range. Some examples of medications that might cause this are beta blockers, ACE inhibitors, and nitrates. Infections of the blood, called *sepsis,* can cause the blood vessels to dilate, reducing the blood pressure.

The treatment for low blood pressure depends on the cause. Heart problems like muscle inflammation or infection can be treated. Blocked arteries can be bypassed, irregular heartbeats can be controlled by medication or a pacemaker, and dysfunctional heart valves can be repaired or replaced. Infections can be treated with antibiotics. Sometimes all that is necessary is for the doctor to adjust your medication.

## 89. What is pulmonary edema?

Pulmonary edema is a serious medical condition. Sometimes called pulmonary congestion or water on the lung, *pulmonary edema* is an excess accumulation of water in the lung tissues that results in the lungs not functioning properly. While pulmonary edema can result from a direct injury to the lung, it is commonly caused by heart failure. When the heart is no longer effective in pumping blood away from the heart, the blood pressure in the lungs increases. The increased blood pressure causes fluid to leak out of the pulmonary veins and into the lung. This fluid in the lung then

*Untreated pulmonary edema can be fatal.*

becomes a barrier to normal oxygen exchange, resulting in shortness of breath. When severe, pulmonary edema can lead to respiratory distress and failure. Untreated pulmonary edema can be fatal.

**Causes of pulmonary edema** The final common pathway of pulmonary edema is fluid leaking from the blood vessels in the lung to the tissues of the lung itself. Fluid can leak from the blood vessels for two main reasons:

1. The blood vessels become injured through trauma, toxic exposure, or infection. The injured blood vessel then leaks fluid into the lung.
2. An increase of blood pressure in the vessels exceeds the blood vessels' ability to contain the fluid, and so the fluid leaks out of the vessels and into the lungs.

Situations that can result in increased blood pressure in the blood vessels of the lung include:

- Complications of a heart attack
- Malfunctioning heart valves
- Cardiomyopathy
- Increased fluid in the blood vessels due to renal failure

Situations that can result in injury to the blood vessels in the lung include:

- Toxins such as poisonous gases
- Excess heat, such as when a patient is in a house fire and inhales the superheated air
- Severe viral and bacterial infections of the lung

**Treatment of pulmonary edema** Like other diseases, the best treatment is fixing the underlying problem, such as lung infection, heart attack, or excessive fluid build-up in the body due to kidney disease. However, this may be difficult or impossible to accomplish in the short run. In an emergency, physicians will treat pulmonary edema by trying to increase the amount of oxygen in the lungs, decrease the blood pressure in the lungs, and decrease the water in the lungs.

An increase of oxygen can be accomplished by giving the patient oxygen by nasal cannula, oxygen mask, or endotracheal intubation. Blood pressure in the lungs can be decreased through the use of diuretics and blood pressure–lowering medication, such as beta blockers, ACE inhibitors, or nitrate medications such as nitroglycerin. When effectively treated, pulmonary edema can resolve in a few hours, without damage to the lungs.

Victoria's comment:

*I've had pulmonary edema in the past. I was very short of breath and felt like I was drowning. I had to go to the emergency room and get treated with oxygen, diuretics, and nitroglycerin paste. Despite what Dr. Quinn writes here, it took most of a day for my breathing to get back to normal, and I had to be admitted to the intensive care unit.*

## 90. What is sleep apnea?

Sleep **apnea** is a condition characterized by episodes of stopped breathing during sleep. In normal conditions, the muscles of the upper part of the throat keep this passage open to allow air to flow into the lungs. These muscles usually relax during sleep, but the passage remains open enough to permit the flow of air. Some individuals have a narrower passage and during sleep, relaxation of these muscles causes the passage to close

**Apnea**

An episode of stopped breathing.

*119*

and air cannot get into the lungs. Loud snoring and labored breathing occur. When complete blockage of the airway occurs, air cannot reach the lungs.

In deep sleep, patients with sleep apnea can stop breathing for a period of time (often more than 10 seconds). These periods of lack of breathing, called *apneas*, are followed by sudden attempts to breathe. These attempts are accompanied by a change to a lighter stage of sleep. The result is fragmented sleep that is not restful, leading to excessive daytime drowsiness. Many patients are not aware of these "apneic" episodes, but bed partners can become concerned. The bed partner's concern is often why a patient will come to see the doctor.

The classic picture of obstructive sleep apnea includes episodes of heavy snoring that begin soon after falling asleep. The snoring proceeds at a regular pace for a period of time, often becoming louder, but is then interrupted by a long silent period during which no breathing is taking place (apnea). The apnea is then interrupted by a loud snort and gasp and the snoring returns to its regular pace. This behavior recurs frequently throughout the night.

**Hypoxia**

A low oxygen level in the blood caused by decreased breathing or impaired lung function.

During the apneas, the oxygen level in the blood falls. Persistent low levels of oxygen called **hypoxia** may cause many of the daytime symptoms. If the condition is severe enough, pulmonary hypertension may develop, leading to right-sided heart failure (or **cor pulmonale**).

**Cor pulmonale**

A disease state that is characterized by an enlarged right ventricle and right-sided heart failure; a result of a lung disease.

Sleep apnea occurs in all age groups and both sexes but is more common in men. Older obese men seem to be at higher risk, though as many as 40 percent of people with obstructive sleep apnea are not obese. It has been estimated that as many as 18 million Americans have sleep apnea. Four percent of middle-aged men and 2 percent of middle-aged women have sleep apnea along with excessive daytime sleepiness.

Nasal obstruction, a large tongue, a narrow airway, and certain shapes of the palate and jaw seem to increase the risk. A large neck or collar size is strongly associated with obstructive sleep apnea. Ingestion of alcohol or sedatives before sleep may predispose a person to episodes of apnea.

**Causes of sleep apnea** Certain mechanical and structural problems in the airway cause the interruptions in breathing during sleep. In some people, apnea occurs when the throat muscles and tongue relax during sleep and partially block the opening of the airway. When the muscles of the soft palate at the base of the tongue and the *uvula* (the small fleshy tissue hanging from the center of the back of the throat) relax and sag, the airway becomes blocked, making breathing labored and noisy and even stopping it altogether. Sleep apnea also can occur in obese people when an excess amount of tissue in the airway causes it to be narrowed. With a narrowed airway, the person continues their efforts to breathe, but air cannot easily flow into or out of the nose or mouth. Unknown to the person, this results in heavy snoring, periods of no breathing, and frequent arousals (causing abrupt changes from deep sleep to light sleep). Ingestion of alcohol and sleeping pills increases the frequency and duration of breathing pauses in people with sleep apnea.

Researchers say congestive heart failure affects nearly 5 million people in the United States, and as many as a third to a half of all heart failure patients also suffer

*Sleep apnea occurs in all age groups and both sexes but is more common in men.*

**Managing Your CHF**

from obstructive sleep apnea. The sleep disorder causes sufferers to stop breathing periodically during sleep, which puts extra strain on the heart and can prompt potentially dangerous surges in blood pressure and heart rates. Studies on experimental animals have shown that, in the absence of any other variable, obstructive sleep apnea results in left ventricular systolic and diastolic dysfunction. Sleep apnea has been associated with poorer survival in patients with congestive heart failure.

Targeting a common sleep disorder with treatment not only helps people with heart failure sleep better, it can make their hearts healthier. The Canadian Positive Airway Pressure study, called CANPAP, published in 2005, shows that people who suffer from both congestive heart failure and obstructive sleep apnea can benefit from a nighttime therapy known as *continuous positive airway pressure* (CPAP).

A masklike device worn over the nose at night that provides CPAP is an effective treatment for sleep apnea. Studies have shown that when CPAP is used on patients with sleep apnea and heart failure, they may experience not only improvements in episodes of sleep apnea, but also a decrease in blood pressure and irregular heart rhythms as well as an improved ejection fraction. Some experts also suggest oxygen therapy or the asthma drug theophylline for this condition.

Because obstructive sleep apnea is so prevalent among people with congestive heart failure, researchers say the use of CPAP could be an important addition to conventional drug-based therapy for congestive heart failure. There needs to be a greater awareness among doctors about the role obstructive sleep apnea plays in congestive heart failure. If you, or your bed partner, are aware of symptoms of heavy snoring, periods of not breathing, or awakening frequently in the night with a choking sensation, you should discuss these episodes with your physician and explore the possibility of sleep apnea.

If CPAP isn't effective or isn't tolerated by the patient, surgery can be performed on the mouth and throat to open the air passages and decrease or eliminate episodes of apnea.

## 91. Are blood clots in the leg common in patients with CHF?

Yes, patients with CHF do have a higher rate of blood clots in the leg. This condition is called *deep venous thrombosis* (DVT). Under normal circumstances, clot formation is a natural process designed to prevent blood loss at the site of a wound. It involves the production of a threadlike material called *fibrin*, which forms a meshwork at the site of the wound. Blood cells called *platelets* are attracted to the fibrin, then clump together to form a clot (also called a *thrombus*).

Blood clots form in the legs of CHF patients because of several factors. These include:

- Increases in the levels of blood-clotting factors, making the blood more likely to clot (a condition called *hypercoagulability*)
- Poor blood circulation, causing the blood to "pool" in the veins of the legs
- An injury to the protective lining of the vein

*Blood clots in
the leg are
serious.*

Some medical conditions that can change these factors
and increase the risk of blood clots in the leg include:

- Congestive heart failure
- Being immobilized or living too sedentary a life
- Emphysema or COPD
- Recent surgical procedures, especially orthopedic
  procedures like hip replacement surgery
- Broken bones and other traumatic injuries
- Cancer

Blood clots in the leg are serious. They cause pain,
swelling, and make walking difficult. However, the
most serious complication of a blood clot in the leg is a
pulmonary embolism. A *pulmonary embolism* is a blood
clot in the lung. When the blood clot in the leg gets big
enough, it can break off and flow up the veins in the leg
and eventually get caught in the lung. If the clot is
small, it will cause chest pain and shortness of breath.
If it is large, it can cause severe shortness of breath, low
blood pressure, and even death.

Most doctors will try to keep the clot from occurring in
the first place by avoiding risk factors, increasing activity, and treating underlying diseases like CHF, cancer,
and emphysema. When the risk for a blood clot is high,
your doctor may prescribe a blood thinner such as heparin or coumadin. When treated with these medications, the risk of blood clots decreases significantly;
these drugs will keep the blood clot from growing bigger. Eventually the blood clot will either dissolve on its
own or it will become hardened and scarred, so that the
risk of it traveling into the lungs is eliminated. Blood
thinners are often prescribed for 6 months or more to
treat a blood clot in the leg. If the underlying condition
that caused the blood clot does not resolve (like immo-

bilization or a broken leg), then the patient may have to take the blood thinners for the rest of his or her life.

Helen's comment:

*Immediately after the birth of my first child I developed a clot in my left leg. It was very painful and I was confined to bed rest. The only treatments at the time were (1) complete bed rest and (2) application of warm compresses applied all day and through the night.*

*Fortunately today, with the advancement of modern medicine and drugs, doctors are able to prevent clots and successfully treat them.*

## 92. Is depression a problem with CHF?

Yes. Depression occurs frequently in the general population and even more frequently in patients with diseases such as CHF. The worsening of symptoms of CHF has a detrimental effect on the patient's lifestyle and ability to cope with daily living. The prevalence rates of depression in congestive heart failure patients range from 24 to 42 percent. Depressed patients with CHF are admitted more frequently to the hospital, don't function as well at home, and even die more frequently than CHF patients without depression.

Because depression is a disorder that is easily missed by physicians because of its nonspecific symptoms, it should be brought to their attention by either the patient or the family or friends. Common symptoms of depression that should be watched for include:

- Changes in appetite
- Sudden loss or gain in weight

- Changes in sleep patterns (either sleeplessness or waking too early)
- Feelings of guilt, hopelessness, and despair
- Mental and physical fatigue
- Inability to make decisions
- Withdrawal from others
- Lack of pleasure in once-pleasurable activities
- Thoughts of death and suicide

When depression is identified, it can be treated and the quality of the patient's life improved. Treatment for the CHF patient with depression is the same as for patients without CHF. Treatment strategies include psychological counseling, education, frequent patient monitoring, and medications. These have a high success rate.

Victoria's comment:

*When I was first diagnosed with CHF, I thought that I was going to die—soon. I was scared. After a few weeks, I figured out that I wasn't going to die, but I wasn't going to be the same and wouldn't be able to do everything that I used to do. I stayed at home a lot and drove my husband crazy. I was pretty depressed but didn't tell anyone, especially my doctors. I don't know why. After a few months I started feeling better and realized that I could still enjoy myself and while I couldn't do everything that I used to, I could still do a lot. If I had to do it over again, I think I'd tell the doctor and see if I could feel better quicker with some antidepressant medications.*

# PART EIGHT

# *Surviving CHF*

What can I do to improve my
quality of life?

Is exercise helpful for patients
with CHF?

How do I stop smoking?

*More . . .*

## 93. What can I do to improve my quality of life?

Patients who work to control their symptoms, studies have shown, have improved outlooks and fewer symptoms than those patients who just "go through the motions." Speak to your doctor, nurse, and pharmacist. Learn all you can about your disease, what your symptoms mean, and how to treat them. Find out how you can help yourself. It will pay off. Some suggestions of taking control of your disease and your life include:

**Be aware of your body.** A great way to avoid worsening of your symptoms is to detect them early and then do something about it. Every CHF patient should have an accurate scale in his or her house. They should weigh themselves every day at the same time of day. Increases of 3 lbs in 24 hours or 5 lbs in a week should prompt a call to your doctor. Watch out for increased shortness of breath, swelling in the hands and feet, or an inability to lie flat in bed. These are symptoms of worsening CHF and they will not improve without treatment.

**Eat a healthy diet.** Limit your consumption of sodium (salt) to less than 2,000 milligrams (2 grams) each day. Eat foods high in fiber and potassium. Limit foods high in fat, cholesterol, and sugar. Reduce your total daily intake of calories to lose weight if necessary.

**Exercise regularly.** A regular cardiovascular exercise program, prescribed by your doctor, will help improve symptoms and strength and make you feel better. It may also decrease heart failure progression. A cardiac rehabilitation program is a good place to start.

**Conserve your energy.** Plan your activities and include rest periods during the day. Certain activities, such as pushing or pulling heavy objects and shoveling, may worsen heart failure and its symptoms. Learn what your limitations are and *don't overdo it.* Too much exercise or emotional stress can worsen your symptoms.

*Too much exercise or emotional stress can worsen your symptoms.*

*Surviving CHF*

**Prevent respiratory infections.** Although CHF patients don't necessarily get more respiratory infections, they can suffer more with the symptoms than someone who does not have CHF. Annual flu shots and a pneumococcal vaccine every 5 years are recommended. Ask your doctor about getting these vaccines.

**Take your medications as prescribed.** Learn about your medications. Studies show that patients who are more familiar with what their medications do and why they have to take them are more compliant with their doctor's recommendations and spend less time in the hospital with heart failure symptoms. Your physician and pharmacists are excellent sources of information. Many times the manufacturer of the drug has a telephone number you can call for more information. Do not stop taking medications without first contacting your doctor.

**Get emotional or psychological support if needed.** An episode with heart failure can be difficult for your whole family. Many people with CHF suffer from depression; counseling and antidepressant medication can help. If you have questions, ask your doctor or nurse. If you need emotional support, social workers, psychologists, clergy, and heart failure support groups are a phone call away. Ask your doctor or nurse to point you in the right direction.

Victoria's comment:

*This is good advice. When you get sick the first time, you start to realize that you can't do everything yourself and you have to start to ask for help. This was not easy for me. I like to think that I can handle things myself. I started asking for help from my doctors, my husband, my kids, and even my neighbors. I was surprised how quickly most people responded. I was able to get a lot of things done through other people and still do those things that I enjoyed personally. For example, I can send my husband shopping for food, but still enjoy preparing meals.*

*I had to focus on myself more than I did before. I had to think about my diet, my medications, and my doctors' appointments. In the beginning, this made me feel guilty. But I was the only one who could manage these things and I couldn't expect anyone else to do it for me. So now I do it and feel better about managing my disease, rather than letting it manage me.*

## 94. Is exercise helpful for patients with heart failure?

CHF is often associated with shortness of breath and fatigue. As a result, patients with CHF are often sedentary. They sit and lie down through much of the day. They may even be told not to exercise because it is dangerous. This sedentary lifestyle affects your heart, lungs, and skeletal muscles, making it even harder for patients to get around and do the things they enjoy. Being sedentary can also put the patient at risk for the development of blood clots in the legs and in the lungs.

In the past, physicians encouraged patients to rest and avoid strenuous exercise. However, recent studies have shown that some exercise is good for CHF patients and can even extend their lives.

For patients with CHF, moderate exercise may be the best therapy, say the authors of a study published in the medical journal *Circulation* in 1999. The authors' study showed that CHF patients in a 14-month exercise program lived longer, had less risk of heart-related death, and had fewer hospital readmissions than a control group during a 3 1/2-year follow-up. One of the physicians in the study reported that exercise not only improves blood flow in the heart but also increases blood flow to the skeletal muscles. This increases the CHF patient's ability to function.

Another study on CHF patients found that heart failure changes distribution of skeletal muscle fibers. In general, there was less muscle as well as fewer of the tiny capillaries that feed the muscles. When CHF patients participated in regular exercise on a stationary bicycle, scientists found that the patients had an improved exercise capacity and that the amount of muscle in their legs increased.

Similar studies have demonstrated other benefits to regular exercise in heart failure patients such as increased endurance, less shortness of breath, less fatigue, and a higher life satisfaction.

Physicians at Duke University Medical Center studied CHF patients who participated in regular exercise and compared them to similar patients with CHF who did not exercise. They concluded that regular exercise in CHF patients improves survival. These physicians reported that regular exercise in CHF patients was safe.

*It is recommended that every CHF patient enroll in a cardiac rehabilitation program.*

The American Heart Association (AHA) now recommends exercise for heart failure patients. An AHA committee reviewed medical literature that showed that exercise training in CHF patients improves exercise capacity and quality of life. Because all CHF patients are not the same, the AHA stressed that the exercise regimen must be individualized for each heart failure patient and cannot simply rely on heart rate as a measure of exercise intensity. Instead, more complicated tests need to be employed, such as the gas exchange measurements, $Vo_2max$ and peak $Vo_2$, or functional ability should be used.

This is why exercise testing by your doctor is so important before starting an exercise program. It is recommended that every CHF patient enroll in a cardiac rehabilitation program. These programs are able to accurately assess a CHF patient's ability to exercise and to prescribe an exercise regimen at a safe intensity.

## Tips on exercise for CHF patients

Exercising will improve your quality of life and lower your risk of death. How much exercise and the type of exercise you should do depend upon your situation. You should discuss these issues thoroughly with your physician or cardiac rehabilitation specialist before engaging in any exercise regimen. The following are suggested topics to discuss with your physician about your exercise plan.

### For aerobic exercises like walking, find out:

- What tests do I need to take before I begin my regimen?
- What should my exercise goals be?

- What exercises are most appropriate for my level of fitness?
- Are there exercises I should avoid?
- How often should I exercise?
- Should I eat before or after exercising? How long before or after exercising?
- Is it important to monitor my heart or breathing rate during or after exercise?
- Should I change my medication regimen to accommodate my exercise schedule? Are some medications better to take before or after exercise?
- When do I know if I've exercised too much? What are the danger signals?
- Should I be lifting weights to increase my strength?
- What weightlifting exercises should I do?

## 95. I've been smoking for 30 years and have already been diagnosed with CHF. Isn't the damage already done? Do I have to quit smoking?

Yes, you should quit smoking. No matter how bad your heart disease is now, continuing to smoke can make it worse. The constituents of tobacco smoke include carbon monoxide, nicotine, and tars. All of these conspire to cause disease in your heart, lungs, and arteries.

The carbon monoxide in cigarette smoke interferes with your body's oxygen-carrying ability. This decreases the amount of oxygen in the bloodstream and ultimately decreases the amount of oxygenated blood reaching the heart muscle.

*No matter how bad your heart disease is now, continuing to smoke can make it worse.*

Cigarette smoke contains nicotine, a substance that causes the adrenal gland to stimulate the release of a

*Smoking is a risk factor for high blood pressure, heart failure, and coronary artery disease, which lead to heart attack.*

hormone that causes your blood pressure to rise abruptly. Nicotine also narrows the vessels that carry the blood, making your already weakened heart pump against increased pressure. Smoking is a risk factor for high blood pressure, heart failure, and coronary artery disease, which lead to heart attack. Smoking harms the heart extensively. The best action you can take to manage CHF is to stop smoking.

In December 2004, a study was published by the *Nicotine & Tobacco Research Journal* that alarmed physicians. This U.S. survey suggests that despite years of consumer education in print and TV ads and in-office patient education, the great majority of smokers are misinformed about the health risks of their habit.

Researchers found that 94 percent of the 1,046 adult smokers they surveyed believed they were adequately informed about the dangers of smoking. However, many either didn't know the answer or answered incorrectly when asked specific questions about those health risks—most importantly, that smoking increased their risk for developing heart disease, cancer, and chronic obstructive pulmonary disease or COPD.

The survey also found a high degree of confusion when it came to "low-tar" and "light" cigarettes, products that have been heavily criticized because of the suggestion by their manufacturers that they are "safer," even though research has not shown them to lower smoking-related disease risk. About two thirds of the survey respondents indicated they thought these products were less harmful than regular cigarettes.

In light of this information, it seems appropriate to state the risks of smoking here, so that everyone reading this, at least, is informed. Facts you should know include:

- Smoking cessation is essential in preventing and slowing the progression of heart and lung diseases such as heart attacks and emphysema. In fact, in 1990 the U.S. Surgeon General stated, "Smoking cessation (stopping smoking) represents the single most important step that smokers can take to enhance the length and quality of their lives."
- Tobacco use is the leading cause of preventable deaths in the United States, claiming 430,000 lives annually. In fact, smoking causes more deaths each year than alcohol, auto accidents, homicide, suicide, and AIDS combined!
- Based on data collected from 1995 to 1999, the U.S. Centers for Disease Control and Prevention (CDC) estimated that adult male smokers lost an average of 13.2 years of life and female smokers lost 14.5 years of life because of smoking.
- 85 percent of lung cancer is caused by smoking.
- 90 percent of COPD is caused by smoking.
- Using smokeless tobacco in any form (including chewing tobacco or snuff) is dangerous and can also lead to addiction and serious health conditions like mouth, throat, and larynx cancer.
- Herbal cigarettes only switch one supply of tar and carbon monoxide for another. Herbal cigarettes are not a healthy substitute for cigarettes.
- While nicotine can be dangerous to your health, the real danger in cigarettes is not nicotine. Instead it is the thousands of toxins present in tobacco and its

combustion products that are responsible for the vast majority of tobacco-caused disease.

- Cigarettes are *far more addictive* than nicotine gum or the patch primarily because of the way in which they deliver nicotine. Therefore, these replacement therapies are helpful in conquering your addiction.

Helen's comment:

*I was exposed to secondhand smoke for many years while living at home. I grew up in a house where my father and three brothers were heavy cigarette smokers and the house always reeked with the smell of tobacco.*

*My father developed heart disease and lung problems that led to difficult breathing even with the slightest exertion.*

*A massive stroke took his life at an early age. I lost two brothers also as a result of the many years of smoking.*

## 96. How do I stop smoking?

Physicians know that many smokers continue smoking not through free choice but because they are addicted to the nicotine in cigarettes. In February 2000, the Royal College of Physicians published a report that concluded that nicotine complied with the established criteria for defining an addictive substance. Cigarette smoking, therefore, should be treated like an addiction. Like any addiction, stopping is difficult but not impossible. Successful smoking cessation is achieved through education, planning, and support from your physician, friends, and family. Quitting does not usually happen on the first try. Research scientists have found that most people try to quit seven times before they succeed. Unsuccessful quit attempts, while frustrating, are actually part of the process of quitting. For most people, the best way to quit will be some combination of medicine, a method to change personal habits, and emotional support. The following sections describe these tools and how they may be helpful for you.

**Get professional help.** Doctors are trained on how to help you stop smoking. They can counsel you, help you choose from a number of quitting strategies, and even prescribe medication that can increase your chances of quitting for good. If you are not interested or can't work with your physician, the American Lung Association, American Cancer Society, Will Rogers Foundation, and others offer courses in how to stop smoking.

Your doctor, dentist, or pharmacist can also point you to places to find support or toll-free "quit" lines. You may want to join a smoking cessation program or support group to help you quit. These programs can work well, if you're willing to commit to them.

With the wide array of counseling services, self-help materials, and medicines available today, smokers have more tools than ever before to help them quit smoking successfully.

**Quitting "cold turkey" isn't your only choice.** Although some smokers are successful with this approach, medical studies reveal that adding nicotine replacement to your smoking cessation plan will double your success rate at quitting for good. The most important element of the cessation process is the smoker's decision to quit, with the aid or method of secondary importance.

*Quitting "cold turkey" isn't your only choice.*

Talk to your doctor about other ways to quit. Most doctors can answer your questions and give advice.

They can suggest medicine to help with withdrawal. Some of these medications require a doctor's prescription; others can be purchased over the counter.

**Join a quit smoking (smoking cessation) program.** How do quit-smoking programs and support groups work? They help smokers spot and cope with problems they have when trying to quit. The programs teach problem-solving and other coping skills. A quit-smoking program can help you quit for good by:

- Helping you better understand why you smoke
- Teaching you how to handle withdrawal and stress
- Teaching you tips to help resist the urge to smoke

A review of smoking cessation products and services found that smokers are up to four times more likely to stop smoking by attending specialist smokers' clinics than by using willpower alone. If you cannot see your doctor, you can get some medicines without a prescription that can help you quit smoking. Go to your local pharmacy or grocery store for over-the-counter medicines like the nicotine patch, nicotine gum, or nicotine lozenge. Read the instructions and ask the pharmacist if the medicine is right for you.

**Prepare mentally for your quit date.** You are not alone in your struggle against your smoking habit! Most smokers in the United States want to quit. However, it can be tough and you will need lots of willpower to break the hold of nicotine, a powerful and addictive drug. Set a date to stop smoking—any day will do—but choosing a date will help mental preparation. Pick a date within the next 2 weeks to quit, but don't wait too long!

If you smoke at work, quit on the weekend or during a day off. That way you'll already be cigarette-free when you return.

In your mental preparation, it is helpful to make a list of all the reasons why you want to stop smoking. Place this list prominently in your home (e.g., your bathroom mirror or refrigerator door) to remind yourself why you're quitting. Here are some sample reasons to get you thinking:

- You'll have better all-round health. Stopping smoking reduces the risk of 50 different illnesses and conditions.
- Heart attack risk drops to the same as that of a non-smoker 3 years after quitting.
- The risk of cancer drops with every year of not smoking.
- Live longer and stay well. One in two long-term smokers dies early and loses about 16 years of life.
- Set a good example to the kids (or other people's kids). You don't want to be a smoking role model.
- You'll have lots of money to spend on other things. Smoking a pack a day can cost $1,800 per year.
- Improved fitness and easier breathing will be the results; you'll be able to participate in sports and get up stairs better.
- You'll have a better chance of having a healthy baby.
- Food and drink taste better.
- Better skin and complexion and no early wrinkles will be a result of smoking cessation.
- Everything smells better—fresher smelling breath, hair, and clothes, and no more cigarette smells around the house.

- You'll be back in full control, no longer craving or being distracted when not smoking or not able to smoke.
- Travel on trains, aircraft, and buses will be easier.
- Work will be easier and you won't have to spend so much time outside or in the smoking room.
- You don't want to support the tobacco companies.

**Understand what to expect when you stop.** Most people find the first few days difficult and for some it can be a long struggle, but things will typically start to get better after the third or fourth day. Nicotine withdrawal may make you restless, irritable, frustrated, sleepless, or accident prone but these things *will* pass and you will quickly start to feel the benefits.

**Anticipate nicotine withdrawal.** When smokers try to cut back or quit, the absence of nicotine leads to withdrawal symptoms. Withdrawal is both physical and psychological. Physically, the body is reacting to the absence of nicotine. Psychologically, the smoker is faced with giving up a habit, which is a major change in behavior. Both must be dealt with if quitting is to be successful.

Withdrawal symptoms can include any of the following:

- Depression
- Feelings of frustration and anger
- Irritability
- Trouble sleeping
- Trouble concentrating
- Restlessness
- Headache
- Tiredness
- Increased appetite

These uncomfortable symptoms lead the smoker to again start smoking cigarettes, to boost blood levels of nicotine back to a level where there are no symptoms.

If a person has smoked regularly for a few weeks or longer and abruptly stops using tobacco or greatly reduces the amount smoked, withdrawal symptoms will occur. Symptoms usually start within a few hours of the last cigarette and peak about 2 to 3 days later. Withdrawal symptoms can last for a few days to several weeks.

**Deal with nicotine withdrawal.** Nicotine is a drug found naturally in tobacco. It is highly addictive—as addictive as heroin and cocaine. Over time, the body becomes physically and psychologically dependent on nicotine. Studies have shown that smokers must overcome both of these to be successful at quitting and staying quit. You can roughly double the chances of successfully quitting smoking by using nicotine replacement therapies such as patches or gum. The idea is to come off nicotine gradually by using a low nicotine dose to take the edge off the cravings and have a "soft landing." Examples of nicotine products include Nicorette gum and lozenges. An alternative to nicotine products is the drug Zyban, which is only available by prescription. Although it is proven to be effective, as with all drugs, there is a risk of side effects and you will need to discuss with your doctor whether this form of therapy would be suitable for you.

**Remove cigarettes and other tobacco products from your home, car, and work.** Getting rid of the things that remind you of smoking will also help you get ready to quit. Try these ideas:

- Throw away all your cigarettes, matches, lighters, and ashtrays. Remember the ashtray and lighter in your car!

*Withdrawal symptoms can last for a few days to several weeks.*

Surviving CHF

- Get rid of the smell of tobacco in your home and other places where you once smoked. Clean your drapes, carpets, clothes, and car.
- Have your dentist clean your teeth to get rid of the smoking stains.

**Don't use herbal cigarettes.** Herbal cigarettes, sometimes referred to as "smokeless tobacco," can also harm your health. These cigarettes are not recommended as aids to giving up smoking because they produce both tar and carbon monoxide. Some brands have a tar content that is higher than tobacco cigarettes. In addition, the use of herbal cigarettes reinforces the habit of smoking which smokers need to overcome.

**Don't use other forms of tobacco instead of cigarettes.** Light or low-tar cigarettes are just as harmful as regular cigarettes. All tobacco products contain harmful chemicals. Some smokers switch to pipes, cigars, or chewing tobacco in the belief that this is a less dangerous form of smoking. However, such smokers may incur the same risks and may even increase them.

**Consider the financial costs.** Smoking is expensive. It isn't hard to figure out how much you spend on smoking: Multiply how much money you spend on tobacco every day by 365 (days per year). The amount may surprise you. Now multiply that by the number of years you have been using tobacco and that amount will probably astound you.

**Involve friends or family.** If you live with someone who smokes, it will be much easier to quit if you do it together. When expecting a baby, both parents should do it together. One common mistake is not to take the effort to quit smoking seriously enough. Really putting your whole commitment behind it will help you have the right frame of mind to face the challenge.

**If quitting is a struggle, consider seeking out other treatments that may help.** Hypnosis, acupuncture, or other treatments may help some people, but there isn't much formal evidence supporting their effectiveness. Use these treatments or services with caution; beware of requests for high fees or claims of "cures" or guarantees of smoking cessation. If you consider these as aids in your struggle or a distraction from nicotine craving, then they have some value.

**Find a (temporary) substitute habit.** Smoking also involves having something to do with the hands or mouth. Nonsmokers manage without this, so it will not be necessary in the long term. But if this is part of the smoking habit, you may need to deal with it. It might be an idea to use chewing gum; drink more water, fruit juice, or tea; or to chew or eat something (but consider weight gain when choosing!).

**Deal with any weight-gain worries.** Yes it is true; many people (more than 80 percent) do gain weight when they quit smoking. The possibility of weight gain is often of particular concern to those who want to give up smoking. Nicotine changes the appetite and body's energy use (metabolism). However, for a smoker who quits, the long-term weight gain is on average only 6–8 lbs. Keep in mind that this weight gain occurs without the person trying to diet or add extra exercise to the daily regimen. Further, this weight gain presents only a minor health risk when compared to the risk of continued smoking. In addition, improved lung function and some of the other health benefits of giving up smoking are likely to make exercise both easier and more beneficial.

**Watch out for a relapse.** You will need to be on your guard especially in the first few days and weeks. "I'll have just one; it can't hurt" is the top of a long and slippery slope. If you are upset or under pressure, it is really important to fight off the temptation to smoke; don't let this be an excuse for slipping back. You could lose everything you've achieved in a momentary lapse.

**Use smoking cessation aids.** Unfortunately, smoking cessation medications have had little use among smokers. The vast majority of smokers attempt to quit smoking on their own, even though unaided quitting has extremely high failure rates compared to other strategies. Hopefully, with the help of their physicians, patients can employ the effective medications available to quit smoking for good.

There are two proven pharmaceutical aids to stopping smoking: nicotine replacement therapy and bupropion, known by its trade name, Zyban. Nicotine replacement therapies, such as chewing gum, skin patch, tablet, nasal spray, or inhaler, are designed to help the smoker to break the habit while providing a reduced dose of nicotine to overcome withdrawal symptoms such as craving and mood changes. Ideally, use of these medications should be accompanied by counseling, which some drug manufacturers provide by means of a toll-free line.

## Nicotine replacement therapy

Nicotine substitutes treat the difficult withdrawal symptoms and cravings that 70 to 90 percent of smokers say is their only reason for not giving up cigarettes. By using a nicotine substitute, a smoker's withdrawal symptoms are reduced. Now available by prescription, nicotine replacement therapy (NRT) is clinically proven to be twice as effective as the cold-turkey method. NRT eases withdrawal symptoms while the smoker gets used to not smoking and the dose is gradually reduced.

NRT only deals with the physical aspects of addiction. It is not intended to be the only method used to help you quit smoking. It should be combined with other smoking cessation methods that address the psychological component of smoking, such as a smoking cessation program. Studies have shown that an approach pairing NRT with a program that helps to change behavior can double your chances of successfully quitting.

NRT is available in many forms, allowing you to choose which will suit you best.

## Patches

Discreet and easy to use, patches work by releasing a steady dose of nicotine into the bloodstream via the skin. Patches should be applied to a hairless part of your body such as your upper arm but don't use in the same place 2 days running.

The 16-hour patch works well for light-to-average tobacco users. It is less likely to cause side effects like skin irritation, racing heartbeat, sleep problems, and headache, but it does not deliver nicotine during the night, so it is not helpful for early morning withdrawal symptoms.

The 24-hour patch provides a steady dose of nicotine, avoiding peaks and troughs. It helps with early morning withdrawal. However, there may be more side

*Nicotine replacement therapy (NRT) is clinically proven to be twice as effective as the cold-turkey method.*

**Surviving CHF**

effects such as disrupted sleep patterns and skin irritation.

## Gum

Nicotine gum is a fast-acting form of replacement that is absorbed through the mucous membrane of the mouth. It can be bought over the counter without a prescription and comes in 2 mg and 4 mg strengths. Nicotine gum allows you to control your nicotine dose. Learning to chew the gum properly is important. The idea is to chew gently until you get the flavor and then "park" the gum in your cheek so that nicotine is absorbed through the lining of the mouth. Long-term dependence is one possible disadvantage of nicotine gum. In fact, research has shown that 15 percent to 20 percent of gum users who successfully quit smoking continue using the gum for a year or longer.

## Nicotine gum and the patch together

The use of nicotine gum and nicotine patches together has not been widely researched and has not yet been approved by the FDA. However, existing studies appear promising. Smokers in most of these studies use the nicotine patches routinely (over 24 hours) and the nicotine gum as a "rescue" of up to four pieces a day without significant side effects.

## Nasal spray

This is the strongest form of NRT and is a small bottle of nicotine solution, which is sprayed directly into the nose. Absorbed faster than any other kind of NRT, this can help heavier smokers, especially where other forms of NRT have failed. The nasal spray delivers nicotine quickly to the bloodstream because it is absorbed through the mucous membranes in the nasal passages. It is available only by prescription. However, the FDA cautions that because this product contains nicotine, it can be addictive. It recommends the spray be prescribed for 3-month periods and should not be used for longer than 6 months.

## Microtab

The microtab is a small white tablet that you place underneath your tongue. It works by being absorbed into the lining of the mouth.

## Lozenge

The lozenge is like a sweet or piece of candy that you suck slowly. It gives you nicotine in a similar way to the microtab. These are the newest forms of NRT on the market. After undergoing the appropriate testing, the FDA recently approved the first nicotine-containing lozenge as an over-the-counter aid in smoking cessation. As with nicotine gum, the Commit TM lozenge is available in two strengths: 2 mg and 4 mg. Smokers determine which dose is appropriate based on how long after waking up they normally have their first cigarette.

## Inhalator

This is a plastic device shaped like a cigarette with a nicotine cartridge fitted into it. Sucking on the mouthpiece releases nicotine vapor, which gets absorbed through your mouth and throat. Inhalators are useful for people who miss the hand-to-mouth action of smoking.

NRT is generally safe for everyone to use and certainly much safer than smoking. The U.S. Agency for Healthcare Research and Quality (AHRQ) clinical practice guideline on smoking cessation recommends nicotine

*NRT is generally safe for everyone to use and certainly much safer than smoking.*

Surviving CHF

replacement therapy for all smokers except pregnant women and people with heart or circulatory diseases. If a health care provider suggests nicotine replacement for people in these groups, the benefits of smoking cessation must outweigh the potential health risks.

As you can see from this section, there are many types of NRTs. When choosing which type of nicotine replacement you will use, think about which method will best fit your lifestyle and pattern of smoking. Issues you may want to consider when choosing a type of nicotine replacement are:

- How much am I smoking now? Do I need a high dose of nicotine?
- Are my cravings worse in the morning when I first get up?
- Do I need quick relief from cravings?
- Do I want or need something to chew or occupy my hands?
- Am I looking for once-a-day convenience?
- Do I need a rescue medication for "breakthrough" urges?
- Is my skin sensitive? Have patches in the past given me a rash?

Some important points to consider:

- Nicotine gums, lozenges, and inhalers are oral substitutes that allow you to control your dosage to help keep cravings at bay.
- Nicotine nasal spray works very quickly when you need it.
- Nicotine inhalers allow you to mimic the use of cigarettes by puffing and holding the inhaler.
- Nicotine patches are convenient and only have to be applied once a day.

- Both inhalers and nasal sprays require a doctor's prescription.
- Some people may not be able to use patches, inhalers, or nasal sprays due to allergies or other conditions.

## Other smoking cessation aids

Bupropion hydrochloride (bupropion, Zyban), also marketed as an antidepressant, was approved for use as a stop-smoking medication in the form of a sustained-release (SR) tablet. It works by desensitizing the brain's nicotine receptors and has shown promising results in clinical trials. The course of treatment lasts around 8 weeks. In one study, Zyban helped 49 percent of smokers quit for at least a month. In the same study, 36 percent of nicotine patch users were able to quit for a month. When both the Zyban tablet and nicotine patch were used together, 58 percent of smokers were able to remain smoke free for over a month.

It is only available by prescription under medical supervision. Zyban is safe for most healthy adults but there are side effects, the most serious of which is the risk of seizures (convulsions). Therefore, bupropion should not be used for patients with seizure disorders and is not recommended for those with a cur-rent or prior diagnosis of bulimia or anorexia nervosa. This risk is estimated to be less than 1 in 1000 but other less serious side effects such as insomnia, nightmares, dry mouth, and headaches are more common. An independent review by a consumer's rights organization found that when buprorion was used in conjunction with regular counseling, it was at least twice as effective as placebo in helping patients to stop smoking.

*You cannot get influenza from the flu vaccine.*

Victoria's comment:

*I never smoked, but my husband did. After I got sick the first time, he stopped smoking because he heard that second hand smoke was bad for me. He used the nicotine patch to help him quit. He hasn't had a cigarette in 8 years. He said it was hard to do, but wanted to keep me from going back to the hospital.*

## 97. Why do I need a flu vaccine and why do I need to get a new one each year?

Many studies performed on CHF patients have demonstrated that the influenza (or flu) vaccine reduces exacerbations in CHF patients that may result in hospitalization. In elderly, high-risk patients, there was an increase in adverse effects with vaccination (mild fever and muscle aches), but these are seen early and are usually mild and transient. The vaccine is made from parts of the influenza virus and no live viruses are used in its preparation. Therefore, you cannot get influenza from the flu vaccine.

Each year, a new influenza virus becomes dominant and causes infections. As a result, each year the makers of influenza vaccines take the most common influenza viruses and make them into a vaccine. When you are inoculated with that vaccine, you are immunized against those viruses that the vaccine makers felt would cause the most problems. The next year brings a new dominant influenza virus and you need to get immunized against it also. Annual influenza vaccines are recommended for CHF patients.

Victoria's comment:

*I get a flu vaccine every year. Once I got a case of the flu anyway, but my doctor told me that the flu vaccine doesn't prevent all cases of the flu. He assured me that I couldn't get the flu from the vaccine. (I had heard that was possible and avoided the vaccine because if it.)*

## 98. What is the pneumococcal vaccine and why do I need it?

A pneumococcal vaccine is a preparation used to create antibodies to pneumococcal bacteria. When your body produces antibodies to a particular bacterium, it can prevent or at least lessen the effects of an infection with that bacterium. One study has found that the vaccine prevents pneumococcal infection in people with CHF and many studies have demonstrated that the pneumococcal vaccine can lower the risk of complications that can result from pneumonia caused by many types of pneumococcal bacteria. It is important to note that the pneumococcal vaccine is not effective at preventing complications of pneumonia caused by other forms of bacteria or by viruses.

According to the Advisory Committee on Immunization Practices (ACIP), a pneumococcal vaccine is recommended for people who are older than 65 years of age or people aged 2 to 64 who are at increased risk of getting pneumococcal pneumonia because of a long-term (chronic) illness, especially heart disease and lung disease. All CHF patients should receive the pneumococcal vaccine and should be encouraged to be revaccinated every 5 to 6 years.

Victoria's comment:

*I got this vaccine also. Actually, I've gotten it twice in the last 10 years. My internist is very concerned about preventing lung infections. He makes sure that I get the flu vaccine and the pnuemococcus vaccine on schedule. He said that pneumonia is harder to fight when you have CHF and it is best to prevent the pneumonia now than to treat it later. That makes sense to me.*

## 99. How do I make the most of my visit with my doctor?

Studies have shown that patients who are involved in their own treatment plan are much more likely to comply with the treatment plan. Further, when the patient collaborates with the doctor, the patient gains a sense of control over the illness. This has been shown to increase a sense of well-being and quality of life.

If all patients with CHF take an active role in the management of their disease, they can expect to achieve optimal results from medications and therapies and avoid the debilitating effects of sedentary living.

See the following list; it contains information that you should share with your doctor at each visit and questions you should ask at each visit. Before visiting your doctor, review these items and make lists of things you want to discuss with your doctor. Remember, you're both interested in keeping you healthy.

**TIP:** It is a good idea to keep a notebook to write the answers to these questions in. Bring that notebook with you to your doctor's appointment.

**Questions to consider before seeing your doctor:**

- Have I been following my doctor's recommendations about diet, exercise, and medication schedule? (Be honest. If you discuss these issues with your doctor, they often can suggest strategies to help you get—or stay—on track.)

- Have I had any new symptoms (fatigue, chest pain, swelling, palpitations)?
- Am I unable to do something recently that I was always able to do?
- What was my last blood pressure reading?
- Have I had any problems getting my medications?
- Have I had any problems affording my medications or other health care?
- Has there been a change in my insurance?
- Has there been a change in my financial status?
- Have I had any problems taking my medications? Have there been any side effects?
- Have I had any problems keeping my medication schedule straight? Have I gotten confused, taken the wrong medication, or missed doses?
- Have I been prescribed any new medications by other doctors?
- Have I been taking any new medications, vitamins, cold pills, home remedies, herbs, and so forth?
- Have I been doing any more work or more exercise than normal? How did this make me feel?
- How has my mood been? Have I been feeling blue or depressed? Do I feel hopeless about my condition?
- Have there been any changes in my household or family? Any births or deaths, more responsibilities, more work, or causes for stress or anxiety?
- Have there been any changes in my "support network": people who check in on you, help you out when necessary, take you shopping, or just come over and visit?
- Am I still able to take care of myself? Do I need extra help to get the usual things done? Who would I talk to if I did need help?
- When was my last influenza vaccine?
- When was my last pneumococcal vaccine?

*You should take notes during your doctor visits.*

- When was my last EKG?
- Have I had all my cancer screening done lately (such as colonoscopy, prostate exam, Pap smear, mammography)?

**TIP:** You should take notes during your doctor visits. This will allow you to review key information and instructions later. If you don't understand a word, idea, or direction, ask your doctor to explain it fully. For example, keep asking questions until you fully understand the doctor's instructions for taking medications—when, how often, and in what amounts. Your doctor may have printed information or instructions available to give you, so you don't have to write so much. Some patients find it helpful to bring a family member or friend to doctor visits. Friends or family members can offer moral support, help take notes, or ask questions.

**Questions to ask your doctor at the office:**

- What's my diagnosis?
- Is my heart failure mild? moderate? severe?
- Will my condition stay the same or get better or worse?
- Will I be able to do the things I usually do and enjoy such as exercise, hobbies, shopping, caring for the house?
- What is the most important thing I can do to help manage my disease?
- Do you recommend a cardiac rehabilitation program? If so, where will it take place? How often?
- If my symptoms get worse, what should I do? Should I take any medication?
- If any symptoms seem to get worse or change suddenly, what's the best way for me to contact you?

- If I need to go to the emergency room, what hospital should I go to?
- What if the health insurance plan doesn't cover the treatment or medication you're recommending? What's our next step?
- If I need advice on financial, legal, or family issues, whom do I ask? Can this person also assist with finding outside help for household tasks and deciding whether to go to a nursing home or retirement community?
- What will this new drug, therapy, or treatment cost? Will it be covered by my insurance? Will it hurt?
- When should I make an appointment to come back and see you?
- Do I need to see other specialists? Why? What will they do for me? When do I need to see them?

**TIP:** It is helpful when you get home to sit down and review this list of things to do.

**Things to do when you come back from the doctor's office:**

- Review your notes. If there is anything you don't understand, call your doctor back and ask him or her to explain it again.
- Get your prescriptions filled. Call the pharmacist or your physician if there is any confusion about type, dosage, or side effects of medication or problems with affordability.
- Place all your prescriptions in an area that is convenient for you to get to. In this area you should have a medication schedule posted that lists times and doses. There are many types of "pill organizers" available at your pharmacy. If you have several

different medications, you may find these helpful in keeping your dosages straight.

- Make any follow-up appointments or clinic visits as soon as you get home. Place the appointments on your calendar or day planner.
- Post the phone numbers for your primary care physician and cardiologist by your telephone, along with a list of your current medications, other medical conditions, and allergies.
- Call the doctor right away if you experience a sudden change or your symptoms get worse.

Helen's comment:

*This is good advice. When I was first diagnosed, I didn't really know a lot about CHF, so I couldn't ask a lot of questions of the doctor. I was lucky to have an internist and cardiologist who were smart and concerned. They worked with me and always asked me a lot of questions about how I was doing at home and if I was having any problems with my medications and such. Over the years I learned what was important to ask and what things I should watch out for. If your doctor doesn't ask you questions like this, you should be asking them those questions.*

*I first started making a list of my symptoms and complaints many years ago—before it was "the thing to do" when planning a visit to my doctor.*

*Some doctors even frowned or made uncomplimentary remarks about my list.*

*Today, the doctor is pleased to go over my list with me. He now realizes it saves him time, and he feels assured that I understand his instructions. I go home not frustrated or annoyed that I "forgot to ask the most important question."*

*I now follow his advice, stay with it, and in a way, I honor my doctor's prescription to help me get well.*

## 100. Where can I get more information about CHF?

There are many resources available on CHF. These include the support organizations and Web sites found on the following pages. Many more resources are available besides those listed here. Check your local library, bookstore, or the Web for books or go to any of the following organizations' Web sites and search for links or resources related to CHF.

# *Online Resources*

### National Heart, Lung, and Blood Institute (NHLBI)

This site provides detailed medical information and patient education pamphlets that can be printed out. It also provides information about current treatment and ongoing research. There are numerous links to other sites that might be useful for people with COPD as well as other heart and lung diseases.

P.O. Box 30105

Bethesda, MD 20824-0105

Phone: 301-251-1222

Web sites: www.nhlbi.nih.gov; www.nhlbi.nih.gov/health/public/chf

### American Heart Association

The American Heart Association is a national voluntary health agency whose mission is to reduce disability and death from cardiovascular diseases and stroke.

Web sites: www.americanheart.org;

www.americanheart.org/presenter.jhtml?identifier=1486

### American College of Chest Physicians

The American College of Chest Physicians (ACCP) is a medical specialty society of physicians, surgeons, allied health professionals, and individuals with doctoral degrees who specialize in diseases of the chest: pulmonology, cardiology, cardiovascular and cardiothoracic surgery, hypertension, critical care medicine, and related disciplines.

This site provides medical information, up-to-date medical alerts regarding medications used to treat heart and lung diseases, and links to patient support groups and other infor-mative sites.

Web site: www.chestnet.org

**American College of Cardiology**

The mission of the American College of Cardiology is to advocate for quality cardiovascular care—through education, research promotion, development and application of standards and guidelines—and to influence health care policy.

Web sites: www.acc.org; www.acc.org/clinical/topic/topic.htm#heartfailure

**Centers for Disease Control and Prevention**

The Centers for Disease Control and Prevention (CDC) is recognized as the lead federal agency for protecting the health and safety of people—at home and abroad—providing credible information to enhance health decisions, and promoting health through strong partnerships.

Web site: www.cdc.gov/search.do?action=search&queryText =CHF

**MedlinePlus: Heartfailure**

This site provides information on heart failure from the national library of medicine.

Web site: www.nlm.nih.gov/medlineplus/heartfailure.html

**Theheart.org**

This site provides information on caring for people with disorders of the heart and circulation and on preventing such disorders.

Web site: http://theheart.org

**CHFPatient.COM**

This Web site provides information and interactive areas online that help you improve and lengthen your life if you have congestive heart failure.

Web site: www.chfpatient.com

**Heart Failure Online**

Improving cardiovascular health through creation and communication of knowledge is the primary intent for this site. Those working this site are always trying to gather and exchange the latest health information and technology, especially to help individuals with heart failure feel better and live longer. Related to this, basic understandings of cardiovascular function are provided. This site is partly supported by the San Diego Cardiac Center and the Sharp Foundation for Cardiovascular Research and Education.

Web site: www.heartfailure.org

## HeartPoint

HeartPoint has been created by medical professionals to provide patients with a source of credible information about heart disease. Having any type of disorder of the heart can be scary. This Web site provides information so that you understand your heart and how to take care of it with the best graphic and written explanations possible.

Web site: www.heartpoint.com/congheartfailure.html

## Heart Failure Society of America

The Heart Failure Society of America, Inc. (HFSA), represents the first organized effort by heart failure experts from the Americas to provide a forum for all those interested in heart function, heart failure, and congestive heart failure research and patient care.

Web site: www.hfsa.org

## The Texas Heart Institute

The Texas Heart Institute is a nonprofit organization dedicated to reducing the devastating toll of cardiovascular disease through innovative and progressive programs in research, education, and improved patient care.

Web site: www.texasheart.org

## HeartInfo.org

HeartInfo.org provides timely and trustworthy patient guides about heart attack, blood pressure, cholesterol, stroke, diet, and more.

Web site: www.heartinfo.org

## The Heart Center Online

Access these physician-edited patient guides, animations, communities of CHF patients, and more.

Appendix

Web site: www.heartcenteronline.com/myheartdr/home/
splash1.cfm?sp_id=33&T_Id=89&searchterm=CHF

### The Cleveland Clinic

The Cleveland Clinic offers information about heart disease and
comprehensive treatment for patients with heart disease. Receive innovative treatment from the nation's experts.
Web site: www.clevelandclinic.org/heartcenter/ pub/
guide/disease/heartfailure/understanding_hf.htm

### The Mayo Clinic

The mission of the Mayo Clinic is to empower people to manage
their health. This is accomplished by providing useful and up-
to-date information and tools that reflect the expertise and
standard of excellence of the Mayo Clinic.
Web site: www.mayoclinic.com

### Heart Failure E

An online newsletter from WebMD Health that provides helpful
information for patients and their caregivers. The following
URL will allow you to sign up to receive this newsletter.
Web site: https://signup.webmd.com/medtronic/etips/
etip-signup.htm?z=4030_0101_2004_00_12

### Staten Island Heart

The Staten Island Heart's Web site for doctors and patients has
useful information on cardiac care and patient education.
Web site: www.siheartdocs.com/patient_education.htm

### BlackHealthCare.com

The site addresses health issues for African-Americans.
Web site: http://blackhealthcare.com.

### My Pill Box

This Web site helps you to create a medication schedule that can
help you to take your medications more accurately. It also contains pictures of heart medications and information about them.
Web site: www.mypillbox.org/mypillbox.php

### Left Ventricular Assist Device (LVAD) Resources

A doctor's excellent presentation on LVADs in current use.
Web site: www.sts.org/doc/3231

Frequently asked questions and answers on LVAD.
Web site: www.sts.org/education/faqs/faqassist.html

Arrow LionHeart (an LVAD manufacturer)
Web site: www.arrowintl.com

DeBakey's LVAD
Home page
Web site: http://micromedtech.com/

Background
Web site: http://technology/jsc.nasa.gov/successstory.cfm

MedQuest's LVAD
Web site: www.medquest-inc.com/products.html

CardialCare's BCM device
Web site: www.cardialcare.com

Implanting a HeartMate Pump including photos
Web site: www.ctsnet.org/doc/1779

*Houston Chronicle* on heart assist and replacement
Web site: www.chron.com/content/chronicle/
metropolitan/heart/index.html

WorldHeart (see products section)
Web site: www.worldheart.com

University of Maryland Heart Center on LVADs
Web site: www.umm.edu/heart/mcsd_devices.html

VentrAssist
Web site: www.ventrassist.com/product/product_set.html

FDA Center for Device and Radiological Health
Web site: www.fda.gov/cdrh

M-Tec, Inc., desk list of medical device manufacturers
www.mtdesk.com/mfg.shtml

**LVAD Information**
Information on portable LVAD
Web site: www.thoratec.com

## *Resources for Smoking Cessation*

### The Centers for Disease Control
Information and resources on quitting smoking.
Web site: www.cdc.gov/tobacco/how2quit.htm

### The U.S. Department of Health and Human Services
This department offers tobacco cessation guidelines, including the latest drugs and counseling techniques for treating tobacco use and dependence.
Web site: www.surgeongeneral.gov/tobacco

### The American Lung Association
The association provides a smoking cessation resource fact sheet.
Web site: www.lungusa.org/site/pp.asp?c=
dvLUK9O0E&b=44456

### QuitNet
This online resource provides information and forums on learning to quit smoking.
Web site: www.quitnet.com

## *Information on Clinical Trials*

Before an investigational drug or treatment can be considered for approval by the U.S. FDA, it must be shown to be both safe and effective. Typically, this is accomplished via clinical research trials—carefully designed and monitored studies intended to test and evaluate investigational drugs and treatment plans.

People may be interested in clinical trials for a variety of reasons. Some people participate in clinical trials as a way to contribute to medical science and to help doctors and researchers find better ways to help others. Others participate in clinical trials to receive investigational treatments because their illness is not responding to standard treatment. Their hope is that the study treatment—possibly an investigational drug or a combination of drugs—will work better for them than standard therapy.

To learn more about or enroll in a clinical trial for CHF patients, see the following Web sites:
www.clinicaltrials.gov/ct/gui/action/SearchAction?
    term=Heart+Failure
www.centerwatch.com/patient/studies/cat162.html

http://mayoclinic.org/congestiveheartfailure/clintrials.html
www.upmc.edu/cardiology/purple/ClinicalTrials/clinicalchf.
   htm#best
www.einthoven.net/enet0009.htm
http://heart.uchc.edu/research/trials.asp?Therap=Cardiology&
   SubTherap=Congestive+Heart+Failure
www.fairviewtransplant.org/heart/clinical_trials.asp

**Personalized trial notification for patients with congestive heart failure:**
This free service provides you with e-mail alerts when new clinical trials match your medical and geographic search criteria.
Web site: www.veritasmedicine.com/ptn.cfm?did=344

## Information on Heart Transplantation

### United Network for Organ Sharing
Excellent organization for obtaining information and current data on transplants.
UNOS Communication Department
P.O. Box 13770
Richmond, VA 23225
Phone: 1-888-TXINFO1; 804-330-8562
Web site: www.unos.org

### National Transplant Society
The society is a nonprofit organization whose goal is to lobby and support people requiring transplants.
853 Sanders Road, Suite 314
Northbrook, IL 60062-2331
Phone: 847-283-9333

### U.S. Department of Health and Human Services
www.organdonor.gov

## Books on CHF

*Success with Heart Failure: Help and Hope for Those with Congestive Heart Failure* by Marc A. Silver
*Congestive Heart Failure: What You Should Know* by Douglas L. Wetherill and Dean J. Kereiakes, MD
*Heart Failure: An Incredibly Easy Miniguide* by Springhouse Corporation.

# Glossary

**ACE inhibitor** Angiotensin converting enzyme inhibitor; drug used to reduce elevated blood pressure, treat congestive heart failure, and alleviate strain on hearts damaged as a result of a heart attack. They work by stopping the body from making angiotensin, a substance in the blood that makes vessels tighten and raises blood pressure.

**Advance directive** This tells your doctor what kind of care you would like to have if you become unable to make medical decisions.

**Amyloidosis** This is a disorder in which insoluble protein fibers are deposited in tissues and organs (like the heart), impairing their function.

**Angina** A medical term for chest pain that occurs because there is not enough oxygen in the heart.

**Angiotensin** Any of several vasoconstrictor substances that cause narrowing of blood vessels.

**Angiotensin II receptor blockers (ARBs)** Medications that lower blood pressure similarly to ACE inhibitors. ARBs are different because they stop angiotensin from working (instead of stopping the body from making it).

**Aorta** The largest artery in the body. It leads from the top of the heart and travels down the chest into the abdomen with branches to arms, legs, and all major organs.

**Aortic valve** The heart valve between the left ventricle and the aorta.

**Apnea** An episode of stopped breathing.

**Ascites** An accumulation of fluid in the abdominal cavity; also called abdominal dropsy.

**Atria** The upper two chambers of the heart.

**Atrium** An upper chamber of the heart.

**Batista procedure** Also called partial left ventriculectomy; a surgical procedure to remodel the left ventricle.

**Beta blockers** Medications that keep the heart rate from increasing in response to stress. Beta blockers are used in the treatment of high blood pressure (hypertension). Some beta blockers are also used to relieve angina (chest pain) and in heart attack patients to help prevent additional heart attacks. Beta blockers are also used to correct irregular heartbeats.

**Biventricular pacing** A pacemaker with leads connected to both the right and left ventricle.

**Bradycardia** A slow heartbeat.

**Brain natriuretic peptide (BNP)** A small protein that is stored mainly in cardiac ventricular myocardium and may be responsive to changes in ventricular filling pressures. It has been shown to decrease the work of the heart, lower blood pressure, and increase the excretion of salt from the body.

**Calcium channel blockers (CCBs)** Drugs that lower blood pressure by relaxing arteries and veins.

**Cardiomyopathy** A disease of the heart muscle, it has many causes.

**Congestion** An accumulation of excessive blood or fluid in the body's vessels or organs.

**Congestive heart failure (CHF)** A common form of heart failure that causes swelling and fluid retention in the legs and ankles and congestion in the lungs.

**Cor pulmonale** A disease state that is characterized by an enlarged right ventricle and right-sided heart failure; a result of a lung disease.

**Coronary artery disease** A condition in which the arteries that supply blood to the heart muscle become blocked. Less oxygen-rich blood can flow to the heart, making it weak. Severe cases can result in heart attack.

**Diastole** Part of the normal cardiac cycle; the heart fills up with blood in preparation for ejecting it in the next phase of the cardiac cycle called systole.

**Diastolic dysfunction** A malfunction of the left ventricle that occurs when the heart muscle enlarges and becomes too stiff. It becomes unable to stretch to receive enough blood and the heart output falls.

**Digitalis** Also known as **digoxin**. A medication that makes the heart pump more strongly and may also help control certain types of irregular heartbeats. Digitalis drugs are medicines made from a type of foxglove plant (*Digitalis purpurea*) that has a stimulating effect on the heart. Digitalis drugs are used to treat heart problems such as CHF and irregular heartbeat.

**Diuretics** Also known as a **water pill**; a medication that increases the excretion of water and salt from the body. It helps the kidneys eliminate salt and water from the bloodstream and increases the rate of urine formation. This helps to reduce high levels of fluid in people with heart failure.

**Do not resuscitate (DNR) order** This is a type of advance directive. A DNR is a request not to have cardiopulmonary resuscitation if your heart stops or if you stop breathing.

**Dor procedure** A surgical procedure to make a dilated left ventricle smaller and more efficient.

**Echocardiogram** A test that employs sound waves to examine the anatomy and function of the heart.

**Edema** A swelling of the tissues of the body as a result of fluid overload.

**Ejection fraction (EF)** The percentage of blood that is ejected from the left ventricle during each heartbeat. It is a measure of the effectiveness of the heart function.

**Electrocardiograms (EKGs or ECGs)** Tests that measure the electrical waves in the heart.

**Endocarditis** An infection, commonly bacterial, that occurs on the inner lining of the heart and heart valves.

**Endotracheal intubation** This is a procedure by which a tube is inserted through the mouth down into the trachea (the large airway from the mouth to the lungs). It is used to help connect a patient to a ventilator.

**Heart attack** Sudden death of a section of the heart muscle caused by a decrease in blood supply to that area.

**Heart failure** An illness in which the heart doesn't pump blood through the body as it should. Heart failure has no cure, but it can be treated with medications, diet, and other lifestyle changes.

**Heart-valve stenosis** A narrowing of the opening of a heart valve. This restricts the outflow of blood and can lead to heart failure.

**Heart valves** Structures in the heart that open and close with each heartbeat. The heart has four valves that work together to control the flow of blood through the heart and body.

**Hypoxia** A low oxygen level in the blood caused by decreased breathing or impaired lung function.

**Implantable cardioverter defibrillator (ICD)** An electronic device that is placed under your skin and connected to your heart. It monitors your heart rhythm and gives a shock to the heart if the rhythm gets too slow or too fast. The shock is able to change the rhythm back to normal.

**Inotropes** Drugs that stimulate the heart to contract more forcefully. IV inotropes are given to treat severe heart failure and include dobutamine, milrinone, and dopamine.

**Left ventricular assist device (LVAD)** This is a mechanical device, connected to the heart, that aids the heart in pumping.

**Left-sided heart failure** A malfunctioning of the left ventricle that results in the backing up of fluid in the lungs.

**Living will** An advance directive; it tells health care workers about your wishes if you are unable to communicate.

**Medical proxy** An advance directive whereby a patient gives decision-making power about his or her health care to another in case he or she is unable to communicate.

**Mitral valve** A valve in the heart that lies between the left atrium (LA) and the left ventricle (LV). The mitral valve and the tricuspid valve are known as the atrioventricular valves, because they lie between the atria and the ventricles of the heart.

**Myocardial infarction (MI)** Another term for heart attack. See **Heart attack** for more information.

**Myocarditis** An inflammation of the heart muscle. Myocarditis is an uncommon disorder caused by viral infections such as coxsackie virus, adenovirus, and echovirus. It may also occur during or after various viral, bacterial, or parasitic infections.

**New York Heart Association (NYHA) Classification** A classification scheme in which a patient's CHF symptoms are divided into four levels of severity.

**Nitrates** A medication that results in the dilation of blood vessels and a decrease in blood pressure, making it easier for blood to flow. They are used to treat chest pain and heart failure. Nitroglycerin tablets are examples.

**Nitroglycerin** A type of nitrate medication, it dilates blood vessels.

**Nitroglycerin (intravenous)** is the IV form of nitroglycerin and is a fast-acting vasodilator that is often given in the hospital to treat severe heart failure.

**Palpitations** Rapid or irregular heartbeats.

**Potassium** A mineral that works with sodium and calcium to help control normal heart rhythm and water balance. Potassium also helps with normal muscle function.

**Power of attorney** An advance directive. This is legal permission for another adult to act on your behalf, especially in legal or health matters.

**Pulmonary edema** Increased fluid in the lungs. This can result from heart failure and is a common cause of shortness of breath in CHF patients.

**Pulmonary vein** The large vein that leads from the lungs to the left atrium in the heart. It carries oxygenated blood to the left side of the heart.

**Pulmonic valve** A valve with three cusps. It lies between the right ventricle and the pulmonary artery.

**Respiratory distress** A difficulty in breathing; shortness of breath at rest.

**Respiratory failure** A decreased ability to get enough oxygen or inability to breathe at all, it results in a decrease in oxygen in the blood and increased carbon dioxide in the blood.

**Right-sided heart failure** A malfunction of the right ventricle. An inability of the right ventricle to pump a sufficient amount of blood into the lungs.

**Side effects** Secondary reactions that result from a medication or therapy. Side effects of some heart failure medications include headache, nausea, dizziness, and low blood pressure.

**Sodium** A mineral that works with potassium and calcium to control normal heart rhythm and water balance. A high-sodium diet can lead to high blood pressure in some people. In people who already have heart failure, too much sodium may make their condition worse.

**Sudden cardiac death** An unexpected death due to heart disease; a death due to heart disease that occurs within 24 hours of the onset of symptoms.

**Systole** That portion of the cardiac cycle in which the ventricles squeeze blood out of the heart.

**Systolic dysfunction** An inability of the heart to squeeze enough blood out of the heart. It often results from dilation and scarring of the heart muscle.

**Tachycardia** A rapid heartbeat.

**Tricuspid valve** A valve in the heart that controls the flow of blood between the right atrium and the right ventricle.

**Valve incompetence** When one of the heart valves no longer functions normally; either decreasing the flow of blood in one direction, called stenosis, or by allowing blood to flow backward through a closed but leaky heart valve, called incompetence.

**Vasodilators** Medication that widens or relaxes the walls of blood vessels. ACE inhibitors, angiotensin II receptor blockers, nitroglycerin, and calcium channel blockers are vasodilators.

**Ventilator** A machine that can push air into the lungs when a patient can no longer breathe for him- or herself.

**Ventricle** One of the two larger chambers of the heart. The ventricles sit below the atria in the heart.

**Ventricular assist devices (VADs)** These are machines that are implanted in the chest to help improve the pumping actions of the heart.

**Ventriculogram** A test that utilizes dye injected into the heart via a catheter. X-ray images are taken of the dye that outlines the inside of the heart. This allows cardiologists to observe the structure and function of the heart.

# *Index*

Cover photos, clockwise from lower right:
© Andres Rodriguez/ShutterStock, Inc.,
© Photodisc,
© LiquidLibrary.

Figures 1-3 courtesy of the American Academy of Orthopaedic Surgeons.

Figure 4 courtesy of Tomas B. Garcia.